PUSHING
FORWARD

Printed in the United States of America
Published in Hellertown, PA
ISBN 978-1-952481-16-1
2 4 6 8 10 9 7 5 3 1 paperback
Library of Congress Control Number: 2021908243

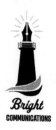

Bright
COMMUNICATIONS

A doctor's story of surviving spinal cord injury
and her action plan for spinal cord injury recovery

PUSHING FORWARD

By Susan Douglas, MD, JD
Neurologist and Spinal Cord Injury Survivor

For my mom, who woke up in the middle of the night at the time of my car accident from 3,000 miles away, came immediately, and has always been there through thick and thin. Thank you for the sacrifices you made for me. Know that I know, and I love you so very much.

CONTENTS

RESOURCES

FOREWORD

Each time I hear a story like Susan Douglas', it feels like the first time. I find it remarkable how survivors of traumatic spinal cord injury are able to return to life on their own terms after such a debilitating injury.

In 1995, anguish filled me when Craig, my very athletic brother, fell more than 70 feet during a rappel off a cliff. He was 45. Craig endured so much of what Dr. Douglas describes in her book: an early hospital stay (lung contusions, broken arm and hand, chopped liver, pain, and confusion) and rehabilitation experience. Craig struggled with the loss of his independence. Yet, within a year, like Dr. Douglas, my brother moved on to an extraordinarily successful life in a wheelchair. One day, when my brother was visiting me soon after his inpatient rehabilitation ceased, Dr. Douglas encouraged him as he watched her toss her wheelchair into the backseat of her car and drive off. My brother marveled at her strength, balance, and grit. Right then, he committed to aspire to that, too.

Sometimes I use a wheelchair for a day in hospital and home—to teach myself some humility and empathy. I have transiently suffered some of the indignities of disability those days. I receive odd looks in the elevator and wonder, *are they pitying me? Or are they afraid of whatever put me on my butt?*

Those days in the wheelchair, a one-and-a-half-inch threshold between rooms might as well be a three-foot wall to get over. My shoulders ache from pushing myself in the chair. Light switches and items on shelves are too high to reach. Inclines and uphill street slants as well. Suddenly I notice how bumpy carpets and cement are. These things and more are now physical and mental obstacles. Of course, with lots of practice, I would probably master mobility within the context of environmental barriers, like Dr. Douglas and all my patients had to do. But after paraplegia or quadriplegia, every daily act becomes tediously challenging,

Today, my brother is a well-known experiential educator and cofounder of Play For Peace. He uses these potentially frustrating moments to teach about disability. Sitting in an elevator in his wheelchair while other passengers stand tall, he might ask the others, "Did you know it's National Paraplegic Week? While I count to 3, please join me by squatting." The other people in the elevator almost always comply, and then they laugh. When someone races to open a door for my brother, he says, "No, thanks. Today, I must open the door for you."

I overhear my brother tell people who are curious about his fate, "Walking is overrated," or, "It's just a flesh wound," or, "Makes life a little more interesting," or, "It would be nice not to have to use a catheter or unknowingly pass some crap or need to use a vacuum gadget to get an erection, but I can ski, play tennis and rugby with other wheelchair jocks, drive with hand controls, ride a three-wheel bike with my arms, and work from a computer. Am I missing out on something?"

In this book, Dr. Douglas offers the newly injured and their family wonderful observations and insights about their physical and mental health after a serious spinal cord injury. Join her on this path worth travelling.

—Bruce Dobkin, MD, Professor of Neurology at UCLA

INTRODUCTION

Each year, 17,730 people in the United States sustain traumatic spinal cord injuries, according to the National Spinal Cord Injury Statistical Center. More than three-quarters of these are male. While the average age of injury was 29 in the 1970s, that has increased to age 43 today.

In 1985, I was one of them. I was 21.

Since my injury, I have learned and discovered ways to survive—and thrive. A traumatic spinal cord injury doesn't change who you are. You are still the same person. You are still you!

Yes, you will face tremendous challenges. Everyday tasks that you used to do with ease will seem daunting—at first. You'll see barriers that other people sail right over—curbs at first look like mountains to surmount, doorways appear like needles to squeeze through, and much-needed bathrooms appear to be miles away. However, you are stronger than you ever knew, you will adapt to your circumstances, and you will overcome these new obstacles.

I have, and you can, too.

In this book, I've shared my story of surviving what should have been an unsurvivable accident and learning to thrive as a paraplegic, in Part 1: My Story.

Then in Part 2: Your Action Plan, I offer my advice, ideas, tips, and solutions—as both a spinal cord injury survivor and a physician—to help you to heal and grow from your injury.

Yes, you've been dealt a crummy hand. I was, too. But you might be surprised at what you learn from your traumatic accident and how far you will go—and grow—from it. You can push forward into the new life of your dreams.

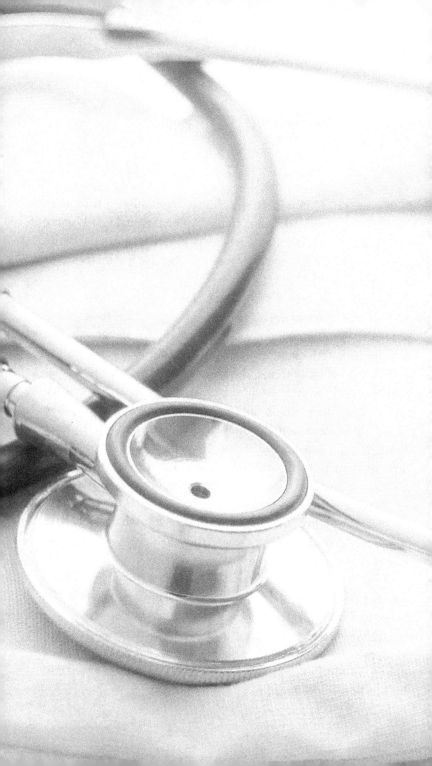

PART 1: MY STORY

Chapter 1: Growing Up in Medicine

Medicine was a huge part of my family's life before I was even born. My parents met while my dad was doing his residency. My mom was a nurse. After residency, my dad opened a practice in a small Iowa town. My mom managed the office. It was a true partnership, and my parents provided excellent medical care for a small community that desperately needed it.

As a young girl, most days after school, I rode my shiny red bike a few streets over to see my parents work. I loved watching them deliver quality health care to the town—as well as to several surrounding farming communities.

My parents wore many hats in our tiny community. My dad quickly became the bedrock and pillar of the community, with my mother by his side. As I grew up, it was wonderful to see my parents interact with the people in our hometown. I admired both of them so much. For many years, I wanted to be a nurse just like my mom. She was a natural nurturer. She checked the patients in, bandaged their wounds, and administered their shots. But as I grew older, I decided instead to become a physician like my dad.

Part of the reason for my change in heart was that of the two, my dad had the more exciting role. I was fortunate to grow up in the era of house calls, and I lived in anticipation of getting to go on a house call with my dad. The phone would ring at dinner time, and I would turn my head in anticipation. Was it another house call? I would run to the car, where my dad would find me waiting and break into his big smile.

"Hey, Susan Mary D, want to go on a house call with me?" he'd ask.

I'd ride along with my dad, joy-filled to accompany him on his next adventure.

Other reasons why I wanted to become a doctor were to emulate my dad's personality, to develop his empathy for patients, and to model his excellence in delivering care. He loved the practice of medicine—everything from delivering a baby to closing a surgical wound.

Because I was so determined to become a doctor, I worked very hard in school, especially high school. I studied long hours for my entrance exams. I knew getting into college and then medical school would be highly competitive. I looked forward to applying to medical school, and I dreamed of the day I'd receive great news of my acceptance.

Most physicians can tell you the story of learning they were accepted into medical school. It's a very celebratory day! After a run to the mailbox, an early clue to your fate is the size of the envelope. A thin envelope is sure to contain a letter apologizing, "We're sorry to inform you that even though you're an exceptional candidate, you haven't been accepted." One day in 1986, my mailbox trip was rewarded with a thick envelope from Georgetown University School of Medicine. I was accepted! I was elated!

Instantly, I was jumping around and running to tell my family the good news. My parents were so proud of me. My brother and sisters were also proud. It was a great day.

After the wonderful news set in, I had the chance to check out the rest of the contents in the big manila envelope. It was filled with all the information I needed to know to begin my journey in my first year of medical school—far across the country in Washington, DC.

Excited and anxious, I packed my bags and got ready for the long road ahead of me. I was embarking on a brand-new adventure in a brand-new city. I was worried about being away from my family, but I was excited to live on my own for the first time. I knew that medical school would be very different from college. I felt like I was growing up and having some responsibility. I was always very conscientious, and I made sure to arrange my schedule so I could get plenty of sleep and have time to complete all my schoolwork on time.

Medical school is expensive. Fortunately, one of my uncles lived in Potomac, Maryland, a DC suburb. He was single, yet he lived in a big house with plenty of room for me. Depending on which route I took, I had a 30 to 40 minute drive to med school.

I was soon a busy medical student. My uncle was busy too, so we were like two ships that barely passed in the night. My uncle was an up-and-coming civil engineer who was responsible for building the Metro subway system that runs through the capitol and connects it with surrounding suburbs. My uncle and I sometimes crossed paths in the mornings, but we definitely weren't accountable to each other. He traveled a lot for work, so sometimes we wouldn't see each other for days. My uncle gave me space to be a young adult, and I thrived with my newfound independence.

Despite my busyness and freedom, I missed my family a lot. These were the days long before social media—even texting, but my mother called me every single night. Not one night went by that I didn't get a phone call from my mom, asking how my day went. If I didn't answer the phone and it went to voice mail, I could always hear a little annoyance in her message. So, the next time the phone rang, I would quickly pick it up, and we would talk about the day, go over what I did, and share how much we missed each other—all of the usual things moms and daughters talk about. Those calls really eased the homesickness I felt being so far away from my family.

I couldn't spend a lot of time wallowing in my homesickness because medical school was hard! The first two years especially are very difficult. I studied for hours and hours, memorizing how the body works, how medicines work, how different chemicals interact with the body, and how one thing that happens in the body causes another thing to change. The amount of knowledge that we learned in the first two years of medical school is hard for people to comprehend, and this is before any clinical training. For every single class, I studied huge textbooks from cover to cover.

In gross anatomy, I dissected actual human bodies to recognize and learn about every single muscle, tendon, and bone. It's critical for medical students to dissect, study, and understand every single part of the human body so that when they are later treating a patient, they know what part of the body is being affected. By the time doctors are treating real, living people, they have already seen all those parts and dissected them apart.

Many people don't realize just how much learning and sacrifice are necessary to become a physician. Most doctors want so much to help people, to heal their suffering, that we want to understand their suffering. Most physicians don't go into medicine to become rich. The truth is, if they did, they'd be greatly disappointed.

I quickly got into the routine of medical school. Each day, I woke early to shower, dress, and drive to my early classes. My labs were held in the afternoon. After that, my classmates and I would hunker down in the library or another favorite studying place to learn and memorize everything that we were taught that day. Our study groups soon blossomed into friendships.

As we formed new friendships, we started to spend what little free time we had socializing. Sometimes we'd go out for dinner together. But mainly our days cycled through class, lab, study, sleep—repeat over and over and over.

It might not sound rigorous, but it was. The hours were long and hard, but once I got into my routine with my supportive study group, it all started to flow. I loved every minute of my new adventure! I was fascinated learning how the body worked. I enjoyed doing the dissections in gross anatomy. I appreciated physiology class, where we learned how the body works. I loved it all—all but missing my family. But the fact that I was loving med school so much made missing them bearable.

Chapter 2: The Accident

On November 21, 1985, I was driving home from working in the lab. It was a crisp fall day. I noticed the leaves were changing colors and falling off the trees. Despite the chill in the air, it was a beautiful autumn day. As I wound my car through the suburban streets on my way home, I thought about my family and smiled.

I was eager to get home to lay my head down and cozy up in bed to get some sleep, before I had to get up to start the same routine over again the next day. I was wearing one of my favorite outfits, which I had bought on a shopping trip back in Iowa with my mom: a turquoise skirt with a perfectly matching vest and shirt, knee-high stockings, and brown shoes. I loved dressing up to go to school. I always had enjoyed shopping with my mom, and when I was living at home, we went shopping almost every weekend. I especially enjoyed picking out my new wardrobe with her for my medical school adventure.

Thanksgiving was just a few days away, but I had decided not to go home because I needed to study for upcoming final examinations between Thanksgiving and the Christmas holiday break. Because of that, I was feeling even more homesick than usual, which I reassured myself was perfectly normal.

As I drove toward my uncle's home along River Road, a beautiful stretch of road that follows the river out to the suburb of Washington, DC where we lived, it started to mist. It wasn't enough rain to get excited about, but it was enough to make the road wet and a little slippery. But I was a Midwestern girl, and I was confident in my driving. A little rain wasn't going to cause me any trouble.

Tired and glad that I was almost home, I had no idea what was going to happen next. I started having trouble holding the car on the road. The mist had combined with oil on the road to make a slick, oily surface. My car was hydroplaning.

My car kept turning to the right. I struggled to keep it on the road, but it persisted, moving more and more toward the right side of the road.

Oh please! Don't let me wreck my car! I thought as my panic grew. My parents are going to be so mad at me if I wreck my car!

Chapter 3: The Hospitalization

I don't know when I lost consciousness. I don't remember being found. The accident was a blur.

What little I do know about being found was told to me later in the hospital. The next morning, about 10 hours after the accident, as rush hour started, a truck was driving by. The driver sat high enough in his vehicle that he spotted my car—high up in a tree in the woods on the side of the road.

No one had cell phones in those days, so the trucker drove to the nearby fire department and told them about the car in the tree he had seen. When the fire department came out, they found my car right away, but they didn't find me right away.

They finally found me at the bottom of a deep ravine nearby. Unconscious. Bleeding. Broken.

The November night had been very cold. When the paramedics tried to take my vital signs, they were unable to get any. I was unresponsive. Dead on arrival.

The paramedics were ready to zip me into a black body bag to take me up the hill when suddenly, I opened my eyes, looked at them, and asked, "Are you here to help me?" I must have looked like a ghost coming back to life.

Things moved quickly then. The paramedics quickly marshaled the help they needed to get me out of the difficult location I was in. They needed to get me to the nearest trauma center, Suburban Hospital, a Level II trauma center in Bethesda, Maryland—fast.

I was clinging to life with several life-threatening injuries. I had several broken ribs, and the bones were like sharp spikes to the organs in my body. I was bleeding into my chest cavity. Several of my ribs were fractured. My spleen was punctured. My back was broken. I was paralyzed.

The first thing I remember is being placed on a gurney and rushed down the hall. When the nurses asked me who they should call, I had the wherewithal to remember that my uncle was out of town, unreachable. Fortunately, I remembered my uncle's ex-wife's phone number. I recited that from memory to the nurses.

My aunt called my parents, who were working in their medical practice—just like any other day. The next thing I remember was seeing my uncle, looking gravely concerned, running alongside the gurney, waving a bouquet of flowers in my face. He is a very successful engineer, and he must have been informed by his ex-wife. He wanted to do the best that he could for my parents—and for me.

Later, my mom told me that she had awoken that night at the same time as my accident. It was her mother's intuition, she believed. We spoke every night, but she had been worried something was wrong because we hadn't spoken that night.

My mom raced to the airport to catch the first flight to come to me. My dad stayed behind to get things organized. He picked up my youngest sister from school, who was 11 years old at the time. My sister told me it was the first time she saw our dad cry.

Meanwhile, I was rushed to surgery to stabilize my injuries. The trauma surgeons hoped that they might be able to return function to my lower back and legs, that I wouldn't be paralyzed. But there was little hope.

The next thing I remember is coming out of surgery. I was placed in a bed that rocked back and forth to keep my body moving and protect my skin. Every 15 seconds it would rock to the left, and I would feel excruciating pain from several broken ribs on my left side. I held my breath in agony. I could barely wait for the bed to rock back on the other side for the few-second reprieve I would have before it would rock back to the side that caused me so much pain.

Around this time, my mom arrived at my bedside.

I was given pain medicine around the clock. It barely touched the pain I was in. I needed so much medicine that one of the nurses was concerned I would become addicted. To me, that seemed to be the least of my worries.

My mom, displeased with the nurse's attitude, called the charge nurse and had my nurse replaced. My dad had arrived, and he was concerned that if we complained too much about my care, the staff would be reluctant to treat me. They knew we were a medical family, and they might have been worried we would cause drama.

As we got reports and information from the surgical team, one surgeon, who had a daughter my age, expressed empathy with us. The doctors tried to give us hope that I would walk again. My mother was determined I would walk again. But my dad and I already knew, and we had lost hope that I would ever walk again. He understood the medical circumstances and the futility in investing energy and funds into ways to walk again. People spend their life savings on false hope.

A stark reality hit me. Growing up, my dad always had the power to fix all my boo-boos. I knew in the ravine that this would be beyond even his medical powers.

After I had been stabilized at Suburban Hospital, I was transferred by helicopter to Georgetown University Hospital—my very own medical school. A surgeon there specialized in putting in steel rods to stabilize in the spine, called Harrington rods. My doctors determined I would need that surgery.

At this point, I was more aware of my surroundings. I could focus more and participate in conversations about my condition and care. I remember doctors and nurses coming in and out of my room. As my classmates, friends, and teachers heard about my accident, they came to visit and offer their support. I felt lucky to be at my medical school where I had so many friends. I appreciated the distractions of their visits from my new reality.

The nights, however, were long, sad, and lonely. I had to deal with a new reality of paralysis. I questioned, *What will the rest of my life be like?* The physicians didn't offer much hope of my walking again, but my mom refused to lose hope. These opposing opinions created a lot of discord and conflict in me.

Even in the bleak darkness in the woods before I was rescued, I knew that I would never walk again. But I was still me. My personality was unchanged. I was determined to become a physician and live an independent life. I just had no idea how I would do that.

One night, after my mom had gone home, I was alone in my hospital room, which was filled with cards, plants, and flowers from friends and family in my hometown and new friends in DC. It was late at night when the phone in my room rang. It was a woman I barely knew from a my medical school class. I don't remember much of our conversation, but I remember the purpose of her call: to introduce me to Buddhist chanting. "Nam myoho renge kyo," she said in a soft, steady voice. "Try a little with me."

I was reluctant, but I went along with her, mostly to be polite.

"Nam myoho renge kyo, nam myoho renge kyo, nam myoho renge kyo, nam myoho renge kyo," we chanted together.

It was awkward at first, but I learned the words easily. Soon I found the inflections in the words soothing and beautiful. She continued to chant with me until I had memorized it and could repeat it on my own.

"Right now, on the phone?" I asked, a little embarrassed to be chanting words I didn't understand over the phone to someone I barely knew.

"Yes," she answered with quiet strength.

I don't remember how long we chanted after that. I don't think it was long. But it made a tremendous impression on me.

She didn't explain how or why I should chant. I just understood that I was supposed to do it. I don't remember how we ended our conversation. She only called that one time. She never visited me that I know of. I haven't heard from her since.

But she changed my life.

To this day, I chant to soothe myself when I'm in pain, anxious, or overwhelmed. After I say a few lines of the chant, I'm elevated to a space where the pain and anxiety do not cause me suffering.

I've since learned that nam myoho renge kyo is a mantra chanted as the central practice of Nicherin Buddhism. The mantra was first revealed by the Japanese Buddhist teacher Nicherin in 1253 CE. It's called daimoku, and the practice of chanting the daimoku is called shodai. The purpose of chanting daimoku is to attain complete and perfect awakening.

I haven't achieved perfect awakening, but the chant has been a reliable friend to me during many times of struggle in my life.

That chant was one of the greatest gifts anyone has ever given me. I hope one day, I will be able to thank her. I am profoundly grateful.

Chapter 4: Rehab

As I grew stronger, the doctors started to prepare me and my parents for discharge from the hospital. The next step, they urged, was rehab.

Early on, I had decided: *Rehab is not for me.*

My injury was in my mid-back, and I had the use of my arms. Other than the traumatic injury I had just suffered, I was healthy. I was young. I was strong.

Even without formal rehab, I was learning to get around well. I spent a month hanging out at Georgetown University. My mom stayed with me the entire time. My dad had to return to their practice in Iowa. My littlest sister returned home with him. Our middle sister went back to college. My brother was in the Navy, and their policy was that only death was cause for leave. He convinced them that it was because I had lived that he wanted to come to encourage me, to help me to believe that I could learn how to get on with life. His short leave of duty with me had ended. Everyone was moving on.

My parents and I didn't receive much counseling on where I should go or what I should do next. In hindsight, I should have gone to a Spinal Cord Injury Model Systems Center. Back then, there were 16 Model System Centers across the country that specialize in spinal cord injury rehabilitation. (Today, there are 14 systems and 5 follow-up centers. Learn more at www.sci-info-pages.com. More about Model Systems Centers in Part 2.) But spinal cord injury was new to me and my family, and neither we nor

Georgetown knew about Model Systems Centers. We didn't know what we needed.

Back in Iowa, my dad asked his medical colleagues for advice. He learned about a small hospital about 40 miles from our house that had a rehabilitation unit for people with neurological injuries, including head injuries.

My mom and I flew there in an air ambulance. I was in a lot of pain on that bumpy ride. I stayed at the small rehab hospital for 31 days, but I didn't like it at all. I was determined to learn as much as I could to regain my independence. I learned how to get dressed, to transfer into and out of a wheelchair, to open a door, and many other life skills. But that hospital was not for me.

I hated rehab. My physical therapist encouraged me persistently, but I had trouble hearing it. Using various strength-training exercises, they tried to strengthen my arms.

"One more, Susan, one more time," they'd coax.

Every part of my upper body hurt from the moment we started rehab until the moment we ended. I might have been able to withstand the pain if I could have rested afterward, but I had to go on with the day after my session. The only upside to doing rehab was that it put me one step closer to getting out of the hospital and back into some sort of semblance of normalcy.

Although the rehab recommended counseling, I resisted it. On their advice, I did go through a program at a counseling center where they electrically stimulated my legs like a bicycle. In hindsight, I think it was masterful of them to get me into a counseling center while I took part in the study to reduce the stigma I felt.

Finally, after a 31-day "sentence" in rehab, I was able to move home. The good news was I was young and healthy, and I had just enough determination to handle whatever life threw my way. I began to view my injury as a challenge.

The bad news is I faced a long road back to a life of independence and happiness.

One of the first purchases was my wheelchair. I dreaded it. Of course, I had used wheelchairs in the trauma center, hospital, and rehab. But I now I needed to get my own chair. Soon I would be saddled with a piece of equipment that would serve as a constant reminder to myself and the world that I could no longer walk.

As my parents and I looked at the slew of chairs lining the walls of the store, I hated each and every one them. I hadn't yet accepted what had happened to me. I didn't want a wheelchair.

Back then, they had manual chairs and power chairs. But there was nothing in between. It was all or nothing. I got a manual chair.

When the salesperson asked me what color chair I wanted, I chose bright, candy apple red. It was much like the shiny red bicycle I used to ride to my parents' practice—during a time that now felt like a lifetime ago. My dad's favorite color was red, but I believe there was something in my subconscious that made me choose that color. Anger. I chose the smallest chair that I could. I wanted there to be as little chair and as much of me as possible.

Ironically, the red color attracted more attention to the chair than I wanted. It was flashy and bright. People could sure see me coming.

Now that I was home, relatives and friends began to visit. They wanted to see me and wish me well. I wasn't ready for people to see me in my chair. "Hide the chair," I began to say to my mom. Before they arrived, I moved to the couch or sat cross-legged on the floor. I asked my mom to hide the chair in the bedroom. I wanted it to appear that I could get up anytime I wanted to.

"You look good," our guests all said. "We're so happy to see you are up and about."

I nodded and smiled, trying to act polite. But inside I wanted to scream at all of them: *What would you know about being in a wheelchair? You try having to get around without being able to walk, and see how far you get!*

But I didn't. Looking back, I was experiencing what Elisabeth Kubler-Ross called the five stages of grief, a pattern of adjustment: denial, anger, bargaining, depression, and acceptance. I was in full-blown anger, but I couldn't let it show.

My first week back at home proved more challenging than I thought. The home I once navigated with ease had become a mine-field of obstacles. When I reached up to get a jar of peanut butter off a high shelf, it slipped out of my hands and onto the floor. I bent down to pick it up, but I dropped it again. Several attempts later, I was able to pick it up. I stopped and sighed. After that experience, I bought several grabbers and stashed them at strategic locations all over my home!

The reality of my new life weighed heavily on me. I never thought this would happen to me. Then when it did, I thought I'd be able to navigate it much more smoothly.

My parents worked hard to help make our home accessible to me. They built an entrance ramp and rearranged furniture so I could wheel my chair around. They made the bathroom accessible by adding a shower bench. We didn't need to do much because I strong.

I had full use of arms. I could do a lot, and I didn't need a lot—at first. I was grateful for that. If the injury had been higher in my spine, I would have lost the use of my arms, too. That hardly felt like a consolation prize, given how hard life was now. I had to relearn how to do regular activities—everything that regularly functioning people take for granted.

As I was struggling with the many physical challenges I now faced, I was also grappling with heavy emotions. My injury was causing me to change the way I think about independence. Pre-injury, I viewed independence as the ability to do everything on my own. Not anymore. Now independence became having the *opportunity* to make decisions for myself—not necessarily doing everything for myself.

Because I was again living at home with my parents, I struggled with feelings that I was a burden. I began to understand how impacted my entire family was. An accident like this doesn't happen to a person; it happens to a family.

At the time, I considered joining a support group. I even tried to find one, but I couldn't find one near me. My family and I all could have benefitted from a loving support group.

Ever since my accident, there had been constant conflict churning just below the surface. My mom hadn't stopped hoping for a cure, but my dad and I knew better. My dad would say he believed I could walk again, but the dejected look on his face belied his words. Most spinal cord injury survivors who regain their ability to walk do so within the first two weeks. I had long since ran out of time.

I pushed the question of walking again out of my mind. Instead, I focused on building strength in my arms and rebuilding my life. I knew I needed to return to medical school. It would be tough, but I could handle it. Nothing was going to take away this chance from me.

Nothing.

A few days later, my dad took me to a car dealership to buy a new car. My car had been totaled in my accident—much like my body. I needed a modified car, one that I could operate with my hands.

My upper body and arms were strong enough that I could get the wheelchair into and out of the car without any other devices, so all I needed were the hand controls to drive. Back then, you had to purchase a car and have it modified to make it accessible. Today, the automobile industry has evolved so much that you can drive a modified car right off the car lot.

I purchased a car, and we had it modified to have hand controls installed. I adjusted to driving with hand controls with ease.

I was grateful for the renewed independence having a car and the ability to drive gave me. Years later, I traded that car in for a modified van with all the bells and whistles to alleviate the heavy lifting of the wheelchair every time I got into and out of the car.

I chose a car that was roomy enough that I could get my wheelchair in and out myself. After transferring to the driver's seat, I folded the chair and placed it behind me. Once I arrived at my destination, I did the reverse and transferred back to my chair to get on my way.

Very soon after my accident, I had promised myself that I would return to medical school. I couldn't let the accident take my medical career away from me, too. Plus, I needed to find purpose and meaning in my life.

I was determined to push forward. After a lot of hard work, just six months after my accident, I was able to return to Georgetown University Medical School. I was the same person that I was six months before. Only I was completely different.

Chapter 5: Return to Medical School

My first day back at Georgetown was just as tough as I had anticipated. I drove back to school in my new car that had been made accessible with hand controls. After much practice, getting in and out of the car and my wheelchair were easy for me now.

Because so many things now were so much harder than before, I knew I needed to make everything I could as easy as possible. Rather than living at my uncle's house and having a 30- to 40-minute commute, I decided to live on campus. My parents had called Georgetown prior to my return and discussed where I would live and what kind of support I would need.

They assigned me to live in the building where Georgetown's basketball team lived because it was larger than other apartments—and thus more accessible. My apartment had an accessible shower.

The benefit to living on campus was it was close to my classes. But it wasn't that close. It was in the lower part of campus where the undergraduates lived, so I had to push my wheelchair all the way up to upper campus to get to class. I was 21, strong, and healthy, so it wasn't hard. In hindsight, all that wheeling was taxing on my body. I wish I had had more information and guidance to protect my body as it aged. (More about doing this in Part 2.)

But I was happy to be on campus and in my own apartment. Although my apartment was far from the sanctuary I would soon learn I needed.

Ironically, having just had a major neurological injury, my first class was neurobiology. It was held in one of the large lecture halls clear across the campus from my apartment. My arms would get a workout in every day, that was for sure. The first day, wanting to hide, I stayed in the back, one of the only places my wheelchair would fit. I listened intently and took notes as the professor spoke.

"Our firm understanding is that nerves do not grow," he said. I wrote that sentence in my notebook. I stared at it for a few minutes. It angered me because I knew that scientists had come to understand that nerves *could* grow—although connecting the growth of the nerve and seeing nerves return to normal function continued to be a problem. I did not appreciate a leading medical school delivering dated neurological understanding to medical students. Even worse, I knew that if nerves don't grow, there really was little hope I would ever walk again. That day, that professor dashed what little hope I had left of ever walking again.

When class was over, I wheeled myself out of the hall toward the double doors to head outside. A gentleman saw me coming and kindly opened the door for me with a smile.

"Are you going to be here every day to open that door for me?" I asked.

The man's face fell from a big smile to a look of shock.

I hadn't meant to be unkind, but those words came from a place of deep struggle within me. I *had* to learn how to do things for myself.

As the man walked away, all I could think was, *How can I get through doors if people don't open them for me?* Suddenly, there were multiple barriers everywhere. Anywhere outside my home, I had to worry, *Where can I park? Which is the easiest door to open? Where is the closest bathroom?*

As my first week back went along, I began to get the hang of where everything was. I knew how long it would take me to get to each class. One day, I cut the time a little short. I rushed to get to class, but the traffic was making me late. I whizzed by a bunch of people on my way to class, one of which was my classmate.

"There's the bitch on wheels," she snickered and whispered

to her friends. Her words stung initially, but the more I thought about it, the more I liked the name. I had the right to be a bitch. I have had a lot to deal with, and no one, no matter how hard they tried, would understand what I was going through. Not only did I like the nickname, I embraced it.

Shortly after my return to Georgetown, I met with the chairman in charge of med student rotations. Medical school is two years of mainly classroom work, followed by two years of clinical rotations, before you go on to more specialty training and fellowships.

"I hope you are not coming here to tell me you want to be a cardiovascular surgeon," he said sarcastically, practically without preamble or greeting.

Part of me had expected people to have more sympathy for me and my plight. But unfortunately, I felt little of that. In fact, the consensus around campus was they did not want me there. They hadn't wanted me to return. Having a paraplegic on campus meant more money was needed to be spent on accommodations for wheelchairs and other necessities to allow me the chance of getting the best education.

Both the school and I were new to this and neither knew what to tell the other. It was all new to both of us. Depending on the individual, I would get different reactions. Some people dismissed the idea that I could complete medical school in a wheelchair. Like waving a red flag in front of a bull, their obnoxiousness spurred me on. I became determined to prove them wrong.

The chairman's sarcasm was no bother to me. I had learned how to navigate this new life with just my parents and very little counsel.

What I wished I could say was, "Yeah, that's exactly what I came to talk about. I want to be a surgeon—a neurosurgeon." But I didn't want to further alienate me from a staff that wished I had never come back. Instead, I asked if we could discuss how to do this rotation.

More than ever, I knew I needed support from people who would understand me. When I had returned home from rehab, I had tried to find a support group. I knew that having other people who had survived spinal cord injuries would help me. I looked again for a group. Again, I came up empty.

So, I decided to start one.

I created a flyer about a new support group, including my name and contact information. I didn't make it specifically about spinal cord injury. I made it more generally about people living after traumatic injuries. I needed to be around like-minded people who understood my situation. Even if they hadn't gone through the exact same injury as me, they could at least understand what it was like to face obstacles completing even the most basic tasks.

A few days after I put up flyers around on the bulletin boards at school, I had formed my group. Although none of them had gone through exactly what I had gone through, they could understand my mental and emotional frustrations.

It was odd for me to admit I needed like-minded people, but I did. As much as my parents tried their best to help me cope, they couldn't understand exactly what I was feeling or thinking.

Our new support group met weekly. Each week, we went around the circle, sharing whatever was on our minds. When I shared my weekly challenges, I was met with smiles, nods, and uh-huhs of agreement. It reassured me that everything was going to be okay. Even if it wasn't, I had a group of people that was willing to support me in whatever challenges I might face.

Quickly, I was adjusting back to life at Georgetown. It didn't matter whether they wanted me back or not—I was there! We were all going to learn how to make everything possible.

After the first year, I had settled back in at Georgetown, and I was ready to move off-campus to my own apartment.

The minute after I left my apartment, all day every day I overcame obstacles and surmounted barriers. Navigating barriers is exhausting! My apartment couldn't be filled with challenges, too.

Over time, we made many changes to my apartment to make it more comfortable. One day when I got back to my apartment from class, a company was outside sawing wood and drilling nails. They transformed the old inaccessible entrance into a beautiful ramp, so it would be easy to get my wheelchair in and out. I couldn't have imagined how much difference that one change would make. Having that barrier removed made for a much better start to each day. It helped keep frustration levels manageable before I even got into my car.

Once you learn how to function comfortably in your own home, you long for it to remain a place with few or no barriers.

After a long day of classes or being on call at the hospital, my apartment was a place to renew and refresh. Once I returned back to my apartment, it was a relief, because it was my sanctuary. I knew that once I went home, I faced so many fewer barriers than I do out in the world. It was—and still is—a dream of mine to build an accessible home that has *no* barriers.

Although I had a lot of control over my apartment and could make changes to accommodate my needs, I had no such control over the classrooms, lecture halls, or labs. I often had to pick myself up, pushing up hard with my arms to lift my bottom up off my wheelchair, so I could see what was on the table. In one lab, when I was too tired to lift myself up, I made it through some projects by using pictures in the textbooks.

In one class, I had to look at tissue under a microscope. The microscope was so high! I didn't want to admit to anyone that I couldn't see in it. I faked my way through that class.

I was more fortunate in gross anatomy to have a chair that would stand up. It was critical really because we were dissecting real bodies. We learned every muscle, bone, and blood vessel. It was intense, and it was a fabulous distraction for me from the very real physical pain I was in. I totally got into it.

Some parts of medical school were such a challenge. That made my successes feel all the sweeter. One day, my professor expected no one to know the answer to his questions. "Where's the prefrontal cortex?" he asked rhetorically. "Or does anyone know how the brain works?"

"I do," I said, then spouted off an answer I had found in our textbook, much to the astonishment of my classmates. My willingness to answer questions in class made it look like I knew everything and was the smartest person in the room. This made me feel good about myself, like I belonged in that classroom.

The professor laughed. Although it was luck that I happened to know a bit about it, I certainly didn't tell him that.

I began to see how my accident and recovery had taught me empathy for my patients. I could connect with them in a special way because I had been through so many medical procedures myself. I remember a very memorable interaction I had with a patient while I was on rotation. He was a famous photographer who had a stroke in the part of the brain that affected his ability to swallow and eat. I did my best to learn as much as I could about him. Although I couldn't magically fix whatever was ailing him, I could at least make him feel as comfortable as possible.

One day, as I made the rounds and entered his room, the attending physician was chatting with a nurse at the foot of his bed.

"This man's never going to swallow again. Might as well give him as many drugs as you can. He's gonna need 'em."

I wheeled myself right up to the patient's bed by his head. He was struggling with the tube that was placed down his throat so he could breathe. I wasn't sure he could hear me, but I spoke to him anyway.

"You have a tube in your throat that's helping you breathe," I whispered in his ear. "I've had one. I know it's really uncomfortable. But it's going to come out. You're going to talk and swallow again. It's going to be okay."

Maybe I had no business saying that to him, but I didn't care. That physician suffered from an ego problem, and if there was even the slightest chance that man could hear what he had said, I didn't want him to give up hope. The man was in the ICU and hadn't had any visitors, and I wanted to be the voice of hope for him. The reality was, we *didn't* know what exactly would happen, and if there was any room for hope, I was going to deliver it. Hope had helped me during my difficult time, and I wanted to do the same for him.

I had wheeled my chair right up to the edge of the bed. Some people might consider that an invasion of privacy, but I didn't. All I could think about was when I was lying in a hospital bed unconsciousness. I remembered what it felt like to be intubated. The air blows in and out of your chest. You have to surrender to it. It's so challenging that most of the time patients are sedated to assist them in surrendering to it. But sometimes when the sedation lightens up, you can feel the air going in and out of your lungs. It's an awful feeling, and one I didn't want to relive.

A few days later, I was making my rounds. I stopped in the photographer's room like I had done every day for weeks. The scene that greeted me was different than what I had ever seen before. Instead of the man lying motionless and unconscious, his eyes were open. When he saw me, a big smile stretched across his face.

"I remembered every word you told me," he said. "I might have given up if you hadn't told me your experience and understood what I was going through."

This was just one of many circumstances that helped me to understand that, in a strange way, my accident helped me become a better doctor.

I also gained the ability to advocate for my patients when they needed one. My parents had advocated for me when I needed pain medicine, when I needed more care, and when everyone gave up on me. Knowing someone was in my corner made it worth getting up to fight for my health and recovery every day. That's what I want to be for each patient entrusted to my care.

After the four years of medical school—long hours of study, countless classes and labs, and dozens of rotations, doctors move on to a three- to seven-year residency program, depending upon which specialty they want to pursue. After all I had been through, naturally I wanted to be a neurologist.

As I finished my clinical years, I focused on trying to be accepted into the best neurology program in the country. In the last year of medical school, I traveled to England to the famous National Hospital for Neurology and Neurosurgery, Queen Square, in London. I learned a lot, and that experience was invaluable in getting the residency I wanted. I also studied at different neurology programs throughout the country to determine which residency was best for me.

My best friend wanted to become a neurologist as well. We participated in the match system, which connects medical students with residency programs. The residency candidates are ranked by the residency programs. At the same time, the candidates rank the programs. For example, if Harvard was my number-one choice, and if they ranked a student like me as their top choice, we would be a match.

My top choice for residency and my best friend's was UCLA. We both matched at UCLA. It was quite a day. All the med students gather in the auditorium. The match letters are passed out that tell you which program you will go to.

On match day, I was still in London. My boyfriend at the time got ahold of my letter. He called me with great excitement to share the news that I was matched to Cedars Sinai Hospital for my intern year and UCLA for the study of my specialty, neurology. I was so happy!

After years of study, taking both a toll on my brain and on my body as I wheeled myself all over Georgetown University Medical School, graduation finally arrived. It was held in the Kennedy Center. The center holds a few thousand people, and it was a long trek from the entrance of the building to the place where I had to line up to receive my diploma. But I didn't mind the fatigue my arms felt after wheeling myself all that way. My sore arms and shoulders were battle scars—symbols of a horrific tragedy that I chose every day to turn from a tragedy into a triumph.

Soon, the microphone boomed, "Good afternoon, graduates and family." The day I had waited for had finally arrived. After speeches and words from other faculty, it was time to give out the diplomas.

Each graduating med student had chosen who we wanted to "robe us"—to place our robes with the medical color green over our heads. I chose the head of the neurology department. I waited in anticipation for my name to be called. As I crossed the stage, the audience erupted in applause. I heard whistles, hoots, and hollers, most of which was from my family who sat proudly in the balcony.

As the chairman placed the green robe around my head, he leaned down and whispered into my ear, "This is going to feel really good."

And it did.

All my physical pain and mental exhaustion melted away in that moment. I wore that robe with pride as I wheeled myself off the stage to join the line of fellow graduates.

"We are so proud of you," my mom said as we snapped more pictures. We went back to my apartment, which was decorated with colorful streamers, balloons, and homemade signs that read, "Congratulations, Susan!" It felt nice to be celebrated—and appreciated. All my hard work, overcoming physical and mental exhaustion, was all worthwhile.

The celebration continued into the night as family and friends arrived to join in the festivities. I was bombarded with cards, flowers, and gifts. The best part by far was my green robe. It commemorated that I had finally completed medical school, and it was a sign I could put my mind on break.

But not for long. Residency was up next.

Chapter 6: Residency

After my graduation, my next big task was to tackle my residency at Cedars Sinai Hospital, in Los Angeles, California. I would be there for one year. The hospital was divided into two towers: north and south. Our sleeping quarters were in the north tower, and the patients' rooms were in the south. It was a long wheel for me in between the two towers.

When I arrived on the first day, I wheeled through the double doors of the entrance into the hospital. Carpeted floors stretched before me as far as I could see. For most people, this wouldn't be a challenge. But carpets make it more difficult to wheel myself around from place to place. This causes me to exert my arms even more, taxing them further.

The good news was my time at Georgetown trained me on how to do clinical rotations, so I had a significant advantage compared with my other colleagues. I had also gained the confidence to ask for additional accommodations, when needed.

I also snuck into an empty hospital room to nap on days I was tired. This way, I didn't have to travel so far back to the north tower. I could get more rest and could care for the patients more efficiently.

But of course, there were also challenges. Because of the lack of time in between patients, I only had time to do the physical exam and write up the paperwork before I had to move on to the next patient. This was different than at Georgetown, where I had the time and energy to spend getting to talk with and getting to know each patient.

On my on-call nights, I would travel back and forth many times between the two towers to care for patients when their nurses would call for me. One night, a nurse, who was newer to the hospital, called me several times to care for a patient. I looked all over for the patient, but I couldn't locate him anywhere. After asking other staff, we quickly realized the nurse had directed me to the wrong place, which cost me a lot of physical exertion and mental frustration. After I cared for the patient, I found the nurse and gave her proper instruction so we could avoid another situation like that.

A family we knew in L.A. located an apartment for me. I was moving into it—sight unseen. Waves of anxiety filled me as I arrived. It's one thing to pick out an apartment myself, but to commit to live in one before seeing it was anxiety producing, to say the least.

When I got out of my car and wheeled myself in through the front door, my anxiety abated. It was a small apartment, but residency brought long hours, and all I had left to do in my spare time was to eat and sleep. So, I didn't need much—nor did I want a large apartment to clean and care for. The kitchen was large enough for me to wheel around without issue. I could reach the stovetop and get into the fridge. I could enter and exit the bathroom and shower easily. I needed a shower chair, but at least the shower was large enough to accommodate one. The laundry room was downstairs in the basement, but I quickly realized that I could put my laundry basket on my lap and take the elevator down.

Although I had little time to socialize, I did have an occasional celebrity sighting in Los Angeles. That was a fun, unexpected benefit to living near Hollywood! One day, I was heading home after a long day at Cedars Sinai. I entered the parking lot to drive home for the evening. The parking staff knew the routine of helping me the best they could with getting me in and out of my car, but it was easiest if I did the wheelchair. Frankly, I had been assembling and disassembling my chair so often it was one of the easiest parts of my day. When I finished putting each wheel and piece of the wheelchair in the seat behind me, I locked eyes with Kevin Costner! He drove by in his car and smiled, with a look of marvel on his face at how easily I was able to take care of myself. I wish everyone made me feel as much kindness as Kevin did that day. Most people I encountered were nice and empathetic, but occasionally, I encountered someone with little—or no—empathy for my situation. Good thing I had not had too many of those encounters, or else it would have cast a shadow of discouragement on my schooling and residency after the accident.

After the year at Cedars Sinai, I got ready to start my neurology residency at UCLA. I soon experienced the same fondness from the chairman at UCLA that I had from the chairman at Georgetown. I received an incredible amount of support, and that level of support continues to this day.

I did my fellowship in neuroscience and rehabilitation. My interests continued to be on the nervous system—specifically the spinal cord. I loved my work. It was a joy to excel in a field I was so passionate about. Plus, I also learned a lot about the intricate working of my own body and about the advances in treating spinal cord injuries. I did research, published papers, and studied neurorehabilitation in patients who had neurological injuries like mine.

Ironically, my studies paralleled the life I was currently experiencing. In residency, I connected to the patients, and I was often called on to give consultations and advice. Sometimes, the attending physicians would ask me to stop by a hospital room. I appreciated this part the most because I could offer the same love and support that I had received when I was in a hospital bed.

Chapter 7: Dating

Will anyone want to date me?

That thought crossed my mind as I looked at myself in the mirror one morning a year after my accident when I was still at Georgetown. For years, I had thrown myself into my schooling, I barely had time to think about dating, let alone show interest in anyone.

No matter how busy I made myself, I still had a nagging feeling in my gut. I wondered if anyone would ever want to date someone like me. If I felt self-conscious out in the world in my wheelchair, surely a date would share the same embarrassment.

It was quite a shock when my phone rang on the one-year anniversary of my accident.

"Hi," said the voice of one of my classmates on the other end.

"Hi," I answered.

One of my classmates had stopped at a pay phone to call me while out with friends. "Want to go out somewhere with me this weekend?"

"Sure, I'll go."

"Want to go to the movies?"

"Yes."

"Friday or Saturday?"

"Friday," I said immediately, hoping then we could also enjoy time on Saturday and Sunday, too. We both jokingly laughed, thinking the same thing.

That date was the beginning of a five-year relationship. It was unfortunate the timing of our relationship, as it was only one year after my accident. In addition to the pressure of medical school, I was still reeling from the injury, and I was wrestling with many emotions.

My boyfriend bore the physical and emotional challenges of dating someone with spinal cord injury. If I could turn back the hands of time, I would have researched Elisabeth Kübler-Ross's five stages of grief. I had buried myself in school and internships. I had no time to unpack the emotional baggage the accident had left me. With the help of a counselor, I could have done the soul work necessary to maintain the relationship and allow it to blossom in a fruitful, successful love.

But my insecurities caused me to constantly test to see if he would stay with me. It posed a barrier. He also became my primary caregiver. Often my care became the focus of the relationship, rather than the blossoming of our love for each other. This all eventually became too much, and unfortunately the relationship ended.

If we had connected later, longer after my accident, and I had been able to go through the emotions and loss that comes with this kind of tragedy, the relationship could have been successful. Although I had my same ambitious, independent spirit from before the accident, the hard reality was that my life had still changed in every way. I did my best to navigate all the difficult emotions that come with a tragedy such as this, but being young and dealing with a constant sense of insecurity proved to be the relationship's kryptonite.

After our relationship ended, a fresh start in residency helped me move on. I became more comfortable with dating. When I told one of my dates about the history of being uncomfortable with dating right after my injury, he said, "It's just another thing, like the color of your hair or what style of music you're into. You haven't changed. Your ride has just changed." His perspective was very helpful as I moved on with dating and relationships. Learning from him that dating was no big deal helped me as I moved on with dating and other relationships.

In fact, I got to be so comfortable with dating that my youngest sister, 10 years younger than me, was jealous that I was dating more than she was.

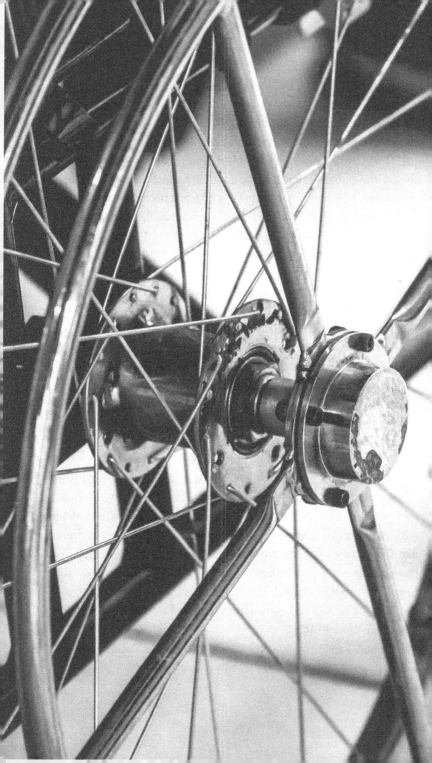

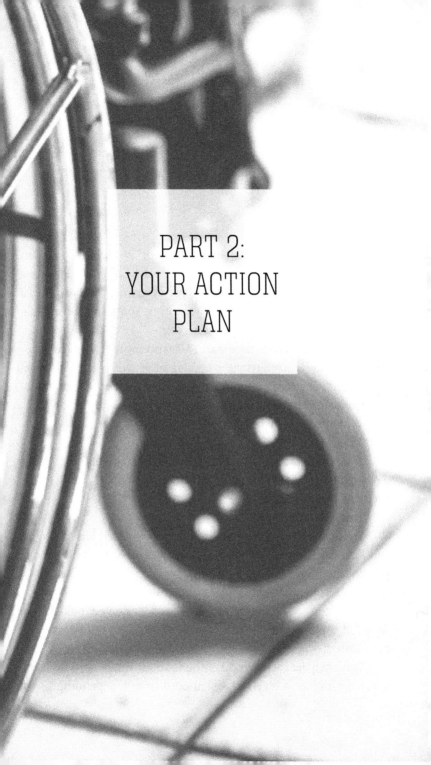

PART 2: YOUR ACTION PLAN

Chapter 8: The Accident

No one ever imagines that it will happen to them. A horrific, unexpected accident that changes your body—and your life—in a way that defies comprehension. The path you imagined you would walk down in life vanishes before your eyes. You might never walk again—not down that path nor any path.

This tragedy befalls more than 17,000 people in the United States each year. They are children, teens, young adults, adults in their prime, and seniors. They are men and women. They are teachers, construction workers, swimmers, mothers, brothers, lovers, and friends.

What will you be now?

That's up to you.

The path you thought you were walking on might be gone, but a new path is being constructed. The fact that you survived a tragic accident speaks volumes:

You are a survivor.

You have overcome something only a tiny fraction of people will ever have to face. If you have survived that, what else could you do?

After your accident, and during your recovery, you probably saw dozens of experts. You were tested, evaluated, poked, and prodded. I bet you know much more about your body than you ever did!

You likely learned a good amount about spinal cord injuries. There are different levels of spinal cord injury, depending upon where the accident occurs:

- Cervical injuries occur from damage to the neck.
- Thoracic injuries occur from damage in your back.
- Sacral injuries occur from damage to your lower back/ tailbone area.

Most spinal cord injuries occur in the cervical or thoracic area. Many of these injuries are caused by diving into shallow water, motor vehicle accidents, falls, or gunshots. The gunshot need not be a direct hit to the spine. A shot to your back can send shock waves that cause severe damage to your spinal cord.

Cervical injuries are devastating. A person who sustains this type of injury will lose function of his legs, trunk, arms, and hands. This is called quadriplegia. If the injury is high enough at the neck, as high as C2, the person won't even be able to breathe on his own. He will need a ventilator to live.

A person with a thoracic injury, like me, might still be able to use his hands and arms, but not his legs. Depending how high on the spine the injury was, the person might have more or less control of the abdomen and trunk. This is called paraplegia.

Sacral injuries are less common than cervical and thoracic. They are generally caused by trauma, such as a car accidents or falls. Sometime this injury can be caused by degeneration through age or osteoporosis. The spinal cord can be injured, but more commonly it's damage to the sciatic nerve—which is the nerve than runs down the back of your legs. Sciatic nerve injury usually causes one leg to be impacted, but not the other.

There's a classification of spinal cord injury by the American Spinal Injury Association (ASIA). There are five levels from ASIA A, when you have complete loss of function, all the way through to ASIA E, where you have some function.

No matter where the spinal cord is damaged, in the neck,

back, or tailbone, your bladder, bowel, and sexual function will be impacted.

ASIA A	The impairment is complete. There is no motor or sensory function left below the level of injury.
ASIA B	The impairment is incomplete. Sensory function, but not motor function, is preserved below the neurologic level (the first normal level above the level of injury) and some sensation is preserved in the sacral segments S4 and S5.
ASIA C	The impairment is incomplete. Motor function is preserved below the neurologic level, but more than half of the key muscles below the neurologic level have a muscle grade less than 3 (i.e., they are not strong enough to move against gravity).
ASIA D	The impairment is incomplete. Motor function is preserved below the neurologic level, and at least half of the key muscles below the neurologic level have a muscle grade of 3 or more (i.e., the joints can be moved against gravity).
ASIA E	The patient's functions are normal. All motor and sensory functions are unhindered.

Functional expectations and prognosis following a spinal cord injury are dependent upon many individualized factors:
- Neurological level of spinal cord Injury
- Severity of spinal cord injury (complete vs incomplete, ASIA Impairment Scale)
- Patient-specific factors
- Age, health, and pre-morbid fitness/function

- Past medical history/co-morbidities
- Associated injuries
- Secondary complications
- Motivation and psychosocial well-being

Most people regain one level of motor function from their initial spinal injury classification completed within 72 hours of injury, with the majority of recovery of function occurring in the first six months. It is also widely accepted that people with an incomplete spinal cord injury can make useful recovery up to two years post-injury, and in some cases may occur more slowly over a longer period of time, in particular with incomplete tetraplegics. Approximately 50 percent of patients initially diagnosed with ASIA B or C Lesions improve over the first few months by one ASIA level (i.e. from ASIA B to ASIA C, or from ASIA C to ASIA D). Ninety percent of people with an incomplete spinal cord injury have some recovery of a motor level in their upper limbs, compared to only 70 to 85 percent of complete injuries. (source: https://www.physiopedia.com/Prognosis_and_Goal_Setting_in_Spinal_Cord_Injury)

Because these injuries are traumatic, they are often accompanied by other injuries. In my case, I broke several ribs and had bleeding into my chest. Sometimes people sustain head trauma, and they often lose consciousness. Spinal cord injury itself is not life-threatening, but so many of the catastrophic injuries that often come with it are.

Most people who sustain an injury like this have a type of pain called neurogenic pain. The pain is relentless and maddening as it occurs at levels where you've lost sensation. This kind of pain is characterized as burning, tingling, and lightening shots. Just a sheet on top of you can cause extreme pain. You also are paralyzed—from the site of the injury down the rest of your body.

You need life-saving medical treatment. Now.

Chapter 9: The Hospitalization

When the ambulance arrived after your accident, you were hopefully whisked to a Level 1 trauma center. Your spine needs to be immobilized and your injuries stabilized. The heroes who come to your aid attend to your life-threatening injuries, too.

Once you are evaluated, you might need immediate surgery. If you have brain injury, you might be sent to a brain injury center. You will likely be hospitalized for up to a month.

You will likely feel extreme pain. On top of this, the pain is refractory to most types of treatment. You just have to wait for your brain to get used to the pain. Somehow, you become naturally distracted. The pain is still there, but it doesn't bother you as much. It helps to add to this distraction with things like meditation. Whatever works for you to distract yourself from this pain, do it.

As your brain begins to be able to process all that is happening to you, the shock will hit like a falling piano. The loss you feel will be unlike anything you ever imagined.

Depending on your personality, stage of life, and support system, you will react differently. A 21-year-old just starting life will respond differently than a 75-year-old grandparent.

But no matter who you are, you are about to experience Elisabeth Kübler-Ross's five stages of grief, a pattern of adjustment: denial, anger, bargaining, depression, and acceptance. Lean into them. It will be hard, but it's vital to returning to a well-adjusted, happy life.

Chapter 10: Rehab

During your hospital stay, your physicians will talk with you about the next step. Do you want to go to rehab? Would you consider a Model Systems Center?

Please consider the latter.

As I mentioned in Part 1, there are currently 14 Model Systems Centers in the United States. I did not go to one. I wish I had. Do as I say, not as I did! Because there are only 14 Model Systems Centers, there might not be one near your home. They often can accommodate patients' families with apartments to live in during your hospital stay.

At the Model Systems Center, you'll receive intensive therapy and counseling from occupational therapists, physical therapists, rehab physicians, and neuropsychologists—all of whom specialize in and are the top experts in treating people like you who have sustained traumatic spinal cord injury. You can attend classes on spinal cord injury recovery. They will teach you valuable life skills, including how to transfer from a wheelchair to a toilet, shower bench, chair, or bed. They'll help you brush your teeth, get dressed, and eat. They'll help you exercise your body, rebuild your strength, and learn efficient, effective, safe ways to maximize the use of the parts of your body still functioning. They'll also help you pick out the most appropriate wheelchair, which you'll need when you go home.

Because you will be sitting or lying down, it causes new challenges for your skin. Being in one place for too long puts undue pressure on your skin. This can cause skin to break down and form sores, called bedsores or pressure sores. They are an injury to the skin and underlying tissue. They can range from mild reddening of the skin to severe tissue damage and sometimes infection that extends into muscle and bone. Bedsores occur especially over bony surfaces, such as the inner or outer ankle, knee, and low back/sacrum.

They are classified into four stages:

- Stage 1: Sores that are not open wounds. The skin may be painful, but it has no breaks or tears. The skin is reddened and does not blanch when you press your finger on it. In a dark-skinned person, the area may appear to be a different color than the surrounding skin, but it might not look red. Skin temperature might be warmer. Skin might feel either firmer or softer than the area around it. If you see this type of sore, call your doctor and ask for a referral to a wound- care specialist. You might have a deep tissue injury that can't be seen.

- Stage 2: The skin breaks open, wears away, or forms an ulcer. The sore expands into deeper layers of skin. It can look like a scrape, blister, or shallow crater in the skin. Sometimes this looks like a blister filled with clear fluid. At this stage, some skin may be damaged beyond repair. You should consult a wound-care specialist.

- Stage 3: The sore gets worse and extends into the tissue beneath the skin, forming a bigger crater. Fat may show in the sore, but not muscle, tendon, or bone.

- Stage 4: The pressure injury is very deep, reaching into muscle and bone, causing extensive damage. Damage to deeper tissues, tendons, and joints may occur.

In stages 3 or 4, serious complications such as infection of the bone (osteomyelitis) or blood (sepsis) can occur if pressure injuries progress. By the time you see a stage 1 sore, you really already have stage 4 injury, but if you attend to it quickly, with the help of a wound-care specialist, you can avoid serious complications and surgery. Sometimes, a deep injury is suspected when there isn't an open wound but the tissue beneath the skin has been damaged.

For the most part, these sores aren't painful. You might feel a little irritation, but the lack of pain can let them grow unnoticed.

The doctors and nurses at the Model Systems Center or rehab will teach you how to care for your skin. Proper skin care includes:

- Wash with a gentle soap, such as Dove.

- Moisturize with a creamy moisturizer, such as Cetaphil.

- Every 15 minutes, do lifts. The average non-neurologically injured person makes unconscious adjustments around every 15 minutes, shifting in her seat or standing up from his desk. You can't do that, so you need to remind yourself to lift your bottom up off your chair. This protects your skin.

- Every day, inspect your skin. Use a long-handled, bendable mirror to check your back and the backs of your legs. If you can, ask a family member or friend to help. I do this during my shower routine.

- If you see a sore, get medical attention right away. The worse the sore becomes, the longer the recovery downtime will be.

More than ever, your body needs the best food and fuel you can eat to heal and recover. Talk with your doctors about eating well. Proper nutrition helps with everything. It helps skin, bowel program, energy, and mood. My palate has always been to gravitate to good foods like fruit, salad, and smoothies. I don't eat a lot of meat.

Control your weight as best you can. The more weight you carry, the harder it is to lift off your seat and transfer from your wheelchair to where you want to go. It's also harder for other people to care for you.

You can get weighed at the doctor or hospital, where you can roll onto a scale and get weighed. In time, you will be so in tune with your body that you can tell when your body isn't looking or feeling the way you want it to look and feel.

Most people who sustain spinal cord injury lose bowel function. In the Model Systems Center, you'll learn a bowel and bladder program. Your body still produces urine and stool.

For the bladder, you need to catheterize yourself. If you have the dexterity, it's best to straight catheterize every four to six hours, depending on how much you drink. Depending on how high your injury is, you'll have different levels of dexterity. Some people have complete dexterity and no problem catheterizing. People with higher cervical injuries will have difficulty with their hands. You may need to have some kind of system that's indwelling—stays in your body—so you don't have to catheterize every four to six hours.

Generally, experts say it's healthier to straight catheterize every four to six hours as it prevents infection over an indwelling catheter, but that's kind of up for debate. What I say is: Your life is hard enough now. Do what's easiest for you. Do what keeps your body healthy as long as you can.

For the bowels, you will need to learn how to stimulate your bowels to have a bowel movement. They won't be automatic anymore. Most people get onto a schedule. Consider taking a suppository to get things moving. The Veterans Administration made humorous videos with helpful instructions on daily bowel and bladder programs. You can find the videos on their website at www.va.gov.

Along with bladder and bowel function, most male spinal cord injury survivors lose sexual function. When a man with this type of injury ejaculates, the ejaculate goes back into the body. Your therapists can help you with these issues. If a man wishes to have children, there are ways to stimulate ejaculation, collect the sperm, then implant the embryo into his partner.

Unlike men who usually lose sexual function, women do not. They are able to have intercourse, orgasm, get pregnant, and even carry a baby to term!

If you choose to go to a rehab center instead of a Model Systems Center—or if circumstances such as your location, resources, or insurance make it prohibitive—know that you can still learn all that you need to do to recover and heal. The doctors' and nurses' expertise at these facilities is invaluable. And they can help you get through the emotional aspect of your recovery, too.

As you process what happened to you and grieve for the life you lost, consider help. Find a counselor you can talk with, and join a support group. You will go through an adjustment period. Let yourself go through that. Allow yourself to feel the shock.

You are likely young. You probably think you know everything. You really didn't want this injury. Allow yourself to go through, *to truly feel* the five stages of grief.

It's important to note that once you've experienced one of the stages, it might not be the only time. Grief has a way of circling around—like a tornado. You might feel denial, then anger, then bargaining. Then something might put you into a tailspin and send you back to anger for awhile. Then, you could skip ahead to depression. People experience these stages in a nonlinear, nonpredictable way. Keep your head above water, stay afloat, and know that each day brings you closer to *acceptance.*

No matter what emotion is gripping you, take heart that you are still the same person. Your personality isn't going to change. Your accident will not take you away from you.

As quickly as you can, develop a fighting spirit. Use every means you have to overcome your challenges and setback. Can you reframe and view your injury as a challenge? Ask yourself, *What can I gain from this?* It might be difficult to hear and impossible to accept right now, but you can, in a way, improve your life.

It is very difficult for the nervous system to recover from injury. If you have a complete injury, it is very challenging to overcome. If you have an incomplete injury, the time period for potential recovery is longer. Don't fall prey to unscrupulous people and spend your life savings on false hope. Instead: Use hope to deal with what's in front of you—hope for your new life. Don't waste your resources on things like traveling to China for a stem-cell transplant. No studies demonstrate a benefit to these procedures. Attempts by U.S.

doctors to duplicate Chinese doctors' results and claims have been unsuccessful. There are data and recommended rules of thumb about avoiding such word-of-mouth offerings for big bucks outside of peer-reviewed controlled trials.

Participation in clinical trials and experimental activities were nascent at the time of my injury. At the current time, there is hype and hope for neuro-repair in spinal cord electrical stimulation and robotics for arm use and walking. But there have been no large studies demonstrating their efficacy either.

Tread carefully if someone asks you to pay a lot of money with the promise that you will regain nerve function.

We've come a long way. There is more funding for nerve repair research now. Back when I was in medical school, it was conventional wisdom that nerves couldn't regrow. Now we know that they can. But we are still a long way from understanding how nerves regrow and how that connects to useful functioning—the functioning that allows you to perform the activities of daily living.

The longer you search in vain and hope for a miracle cure, the longer you will remain in the denial stage. That's only the first stage! You can't move on until you get past denial. You are delaying your progress, healing, and recovery. The quicker you accept reality, the quicker you can adjust to your new life. Deal with what's in front of you at the moment. What's going to come will come.

Before you leave the center, line up the medical care-providers who will care for you next. Physiatry is the specialty that deals with rehab and people who have long-term chronic disability. Another expert you might need is a neurologist. You should check in with your physiatrist every three months or so. As time goes on if you're doing fine, change it to six months. Today, you can do telecalls and check in.

Depending upon insurance, most people stay at rehab or Model System Centers for a few weeks. Then, it's time to return to your old home—or to a new one, if that's better suited for you.

Chapter 11: Return to Home

Once you are ready to leave the Model Systems Center or rehab center, you need to find a safe, comfortable home. Perhaps it's the same home you left. Or, maybe it's someplace new. A few people need to go to an assisted living center. No matter where you go, you will need to make some changes to accommodate your new needs. Here are some ideas.

First, find a way that you can actually get into your home. You might need to install a ramp or use a different entrance than you're used to.

Next, take a spin around your home in your wheelchair. Ask family or friends to move things to create clear paths for you to wheel. If doorways are a tight squeeze, perhaps you can remove the door, remove the door jam, or replace the hinges with reverse hinges.

Invest in tools to make everyday life easier, such as:

- Grabbers to reach high things.

- Holders to better grasp silverware.

- Special cups to use to rinse and spit while brushing your teeth.

- Easier doorknobs to turn.

- Remote controls for TVs, lights, and fans.

- Shower benches to sit on while bathing.

- Mirrors with long handles that bend so you can see your back and lower legs.

- Beds that raise and lower.

- Trapeze that goes above your bed or chair that you can reach, grab, and help you lift up and out of your bed or chair.

- Front-loading clothes washer and dryer.

- Stairlifts to go up and down steps (Though you'll need to have a wheelchair on each level of your home or someone to carry it up and down the stairs for you.)

Soon, you will be ready to venture out of your home—you'll run errands, socialize, even go back to work. Once you do, back in the real world, your day will be filled with overcoming obstacles and getting around barriers.

To cope with that, I encourage you to make your home your sanctuary. Make it as free of barriers, obstacles, challenges, and annoyances as possible. When you come home, you should feel a sigh of relief.

Hopefully, your family and friends have been supporting you, visiting you, helping you, and cheering you on. Not everyone is able to visit hospitals or rehab centers, but now that you are home, hopefully you can connect more with your support system.

Try to get back engaged with your friends. They're going to want to know how best to help and support you. It can be hard to accept help—and even harder to ask for it. But, you are doing yourself a favor to accept it, and likely you are making this adjustment easier for your friends, too. Giving them a way to help eases this for them. The best thing is to be open and honest. Your true friendships should continue naturally, organically. In short time, your friends won't even see your wheelchair. They'll just see *you*.

The hard truth is that you might lose a friend or two along the way. Some people can't understand what you are going through. They can't possibly relate or empathize with you. You don't want those friends anyway.

The flip side of being home is that you are probably being cared for now by family and friends. You might notice your family and friends having emotional challenges, too. Like you, they have gone through something traumatic. Suggest they seek counseling too, if necessary. Realize that they are adjusting to your loss also. They, too, have experienced a loss. The family dynamic changes significantly. Remember to communicate with each other. Give each other space, if needed. Nurture the relationships. Express your feelings—your gratitude but also your stress. Do your best to encourage them to do the same. It's important for everyone to say what they're thinking and how they're feeling, because it definitely affects the entire family.

It's easy to slip into feeling like you are a burden. It's common for people to feel like they are a burden on their families. Try to resist putting this burden on yourself—and on them. It's not your responsibility to fix the family. Everyone's different coping strategies will come up, and they will each deal with it differently. Being in control means having open communication. It can solve problems of the stress and feeling like a burden. You're not the only one who doesn't know what to do.

Important caveat: It's not common, but in circumstances where one person is caring for another, there is the possibility for abuse and neglect. If you are being harmed or neglected, call a trusted friend or family member for help, or call 911.

To help you think and talk through issues like this that come up, consider finding a support group. If you follow only one piece of my advice: Join a support group. It will do wonders for your mental, emotional, and physical health. If you get depressed and fall into negative thinking, talk to your peers and professionals, family and friends—anyone who might help you find solutions. Remember, you *do* have control over your life. Focus on what you can control—rather than what you can't.

In the beginning, I recommend leaning on and depending upon other people. But as time goes on, gradually seek ways to become independent.

Now that you're home, you need to buy your own wheelchair. Yes, this is likely to be an emotional event. You didn't want to be in a wheelchair for the rest of your life. This step means a lot. So much has changed for you. You can't walk, but your wheelchair represents a way that you *can* be mobile.

Your chair will be special ordered for you—custom made to fit your body. The type of chair you get depends upon your level of injury. The higher your injury was, the more assistance you need from your chair.

If you have arm mobility, a manual chair provides a workout, but in the long term, it can over-tax your body. There's technology now, called power assist, that helps you push the chair yourself if you have your arm function, but it makes the push easier. It's less taxing on your arms. As you get older, you'll have fewer overuse and shoulder problems that will limit you. Consider the future, and find a chair to help you reduce the overuse of your body. While you're at it, choose a color that speaks to you.

Consider buying a good cushion for your chair. My favorite is a ROHO. It has 16 small tubes that inflate and deflate, as needed, so the cushion adjusts to your body as you move.

Wheelchairs are covered by insurance. If you don't have the kind of insurance that covers the chair you need, there are non-profit organizations that can help. As your life and circumstances change, your type of chair will change, too. There are lots of specially made chairs now, such as chairs that wheel on sand, uneven ground, raise up to standing height, and more. Most people with spinal cord injury don't use the foldable kind. Most use rigid back chairs that disassemble to get them in and out of cars.

Speaking of cars, perhaps you're in the market for a new one. Consider one that will easily accommodate your chair. You can have an existing car modified with hand controls—or you can buy an accessible one right off the car lot these days! Whichever car you choose, practice using the hand controls and getting your chair in and out before driving solo.

To prepare for going out, apply for a persons with disability parking space placard or license plate for your vehicle. If you are out and see someone illegally parked in a handicapped spot, you can report them. There's an app for that! It's called Parking Mobility.

Now more than ever, you will want to park close to your home. If you don't have a garage or off-street parking, you can contact your city or municipal parking authority or public works department and apply for a special marked, dedicated parking spot right outside your home. Remember to have your chair serviced regularly, every three to six months. Wobbly wheels can cause shoulder pain. Also make sure your tires are properly inflated.

While you can go anywhere with your wheelchair and car, sometimes it's nice not to have to. Those are the times delivery is great. Check around to find national and local businesses that deliver. These days, you can have just about anything delivered, from Chinese food to chicken feed to toilet paper to towels. Although there are more wheelchair accessible taxis these days, there's also a service in every state called Access. It's free or low cost, and they will take you anywhere. You have to apply and have your doctor certify that you need this transportation assistance. The best thing about it is the vehicles are accessible, and you can use it to get around. You receive a card with your own number that you use to make reservations.

Now that you are home and not surrounded by doctors and nurses 24/7, you need to learn about your body—you are the foremost expert on your body. Some common conditions often become secondary complications of spinal cord injury. These problems frequently occur, so keep a watchful eye for them. Call your doctor at the first sign of symptoms.

- Urinary tract infection: These infections, commonly called UTIs, can be caused by putting a catheter in and out. Before your accident, you'd feel a burning or stinging when you urinate. You can't feel that now, so watch for cloudy, dark, foul-smelling urine. You can prevent a UTI by drinking plenty of water and cranberry juice and taking vitamin C.

- Low or high blood pressure: Generally, this can't be felt. It's a good idea to buy a blood pressure monitor and check your pressure daily. Normal blood pressure is lower than 120/80.

- Autonomic dysreflexia: This is sudden-onset extremely high blood pressure that happens to people with T6 injuries and above. It is a medical emergency. Symptoms include blurry vision, dilated pupils, dizziness, sweating, and fever. When your pressure gets that high, you can feel it. Call 911 or have someone take you to an emergency room right away.

- Arm, shoulder, and neck overuse and pain: This is caused by overtaxing your muscles. Try to rest when you can. Choose a type of wheelchair to assist you. Take care of your body as best you can.

- Bedsores: See information in Chapter 10: Rehab.

- Sleep apnea: This condition, which causes you to stop and start breathing in your sleep, can be caused by pain medications.

- Bowel obstruction: The bowel motility is slower, which can result in obstruction. It's rare, but you can get bowel obstruction if you're taking a lot of medication for pain, which can make you constipated.

- Deep vein thrombosis (DVT): This isn't a problem right after discharge, but it can develop as more time passes. These are a problem because you can't stimulate your muscles, especially if you are flying and sitting for a long time and really can't move. To prevent blood clots and to reduce swelling in your legs, wear TED (thrombo-embolic deterrent hose). It's important to remove the hose occasionally. Most people wear them during the day and remove them at night. To reduce swelling, elevate your legs higher than your heart.

- Pain: Severe, unrelenting pain is very common in spinal cord injuries. It's called neurogenic pain, and you get it where you don't have sensation. It can also be called central pain, or neuropathic pain. It's pain that originates from the nervous system. For example, it might feel like your hand is burning or that you've broken your ribs. It's very difficult to treat; nothing works. I have tried everything. Over time, you get used to it. You just deal with it. It's best to find a coping mechanism such as meditation, counseling, or socializing to distract yourself. Although this pain is very resistant to treatment, if you have this pain talk with your pain specialist. This might be your neurosurgeon or neurologist or you could be referred to a physician who specializes in pain treatment. There are drugs and other therapies that reduce pain for some people with neurogenic pain. The only time it goes away for me is when I'm sleeping. As soon as I wake up, the pain comes back.

Although so much has changed for you, remember to maintain your usual healthy habits, such as seeing your doctor yearly, seeing your dentist twice a year, women seeing your gynecologist, and men over 40 getting a yearly prostate exam. Having a spinal cord injury doesn't protect you against other illnesses, such as diabetes, high blood pressure, and cancer.

Chapter 12: Return to Work

Depending on your job, you might be able to go back to work. Or, you might need to change careers. Either way, there are many benefits to returning to work.

First, of course, you probably need to earn a living!

Second, work gives meaning and purpose to life.

Third, most people have friends and camaraderie at work. All of these things are beneficial to you. It's more likely for you to be accommodated at a job you had prior. You are likely to get more support there than starting at a new place.

I encourage you to go to a vocational rehabilitation center. Every state has one. They might pay for some of your home modifications. They help a lot with schooling, tools, and resources to get back into life. (See Resources beginning on page 72 for more information.)

The veterans have a vocational rehab program called Veteran Readiness and Employment.

If you can no longer do your old profession, talk with your social worker to help you apply for assistance, such as social security disability income (SSDI), Medicare, or Medicaid.

You might be ready to return to your workplace, but is your workplace ready for you? Talk with your supervisor, human resources department, or disability office about your needs. Work with them so they can help you.

Businesses have to accommodate you. Buildings built a long time ago are grandfathered, so they don't have to make modifications for accessibility, but most places have to become accessible. If you need special things to do your job, they must provide them, such as a suitable desk or workstation. It's part of the Americans with Disabilities Act. Sometimes, workplaces simply don't know, and telling them will help both of you.

If returning to your workplace and commuting feels daunting, it might be a great time to consider remote work. As I write this, we are living through a global pandemic. More people than ever are working from home. Some love it; others not so much.

When you return to work, day by day, it will feel more normal. Just like when you change your hair, your style, or anything else, people will get used to seeing you in your wheelchair.

The more you access the support groups and different services that are out there, the more support you'll get, and the easier it will be.

It can be hard emotionally to go back to work. But over time, the more you engage with your coworkers, the more comfortable you will become, and the more you make them feel comfortable, the better it will be. My experience was that the wheelchair "goes away quickly." When I was interviewed for residency, two of my interviewers said they didn't recognize that I was in a wheelchair. They were just asking me questions, we were talking, and the wheelchair disappeared into the background.

Chapter 13: Dating and Relationships

As with anything in life, it's all about the people. Perhaps you are single and wish to date. Or, maybe you are dating and want to become more serious. Maybe you're married and want to nurture your relationship.

You are still the same person you were before your accident—a person who needs friends and love. Now you might worry that no one will want you.

It's been my experience that the more you reach out and get out, the more visible you are, the more you will see that people treat your disability as no big deal. It's just a fact about you.

A great thing to consider is adaptive sports. Just about every sport has been adapted. Check out the United Spinal Organization at www.unitedspinal.org. Great sports to try include adaptive:

- Basketball
- Bicycling
- Kayaking
- Skiing
- Surfing
- Tennis

When you get into activities like that, it starts taking away from the stigma that you might be feeling from society. Plus, sports get you into shape! They're good for mental health, and you will make friends to boot!

If you want to date, one option, if it's hard to go out is to try internet dating. Be sure to disclose your wheelchair right away. You might connect with a partner who also has had a traumatic injury. That's a very common situation. You will have a deeply special bond.

A word of caution: It's natural that there will be some caregiving. But be careful in making your lover your primary caregiver. It may be too much. It's important to allow your partner to work toward his/her purpose in whatever he/she is doing to achieve his/her goals in life. Taking care of you can build resentments. I'm not saying he/she can't help you at all ever. He/she can help you lift into a chair or something small, but if you need someone to help you shower and do your bowel and bladder program, have a caregiver do that. Otherwise, your relationship is going to be just your partner taking care of you.

Sure, there are people out there who wouldn't want to date someone in a wheelchair. But you wouldn't want to date them either!

You can have a completely normal relationship with someone, have children if you wish, and a life—just like everyone else.

Even though you have a spinal cord injury, you have control over how you want to feel and what you want to think. I understand if you want to stay in your sanctuary. But don't forget that you can be happy and hopeful about your life. It's only going to happen if you work toward it and want to make it happen. You can reach your goals and have the life that you want.

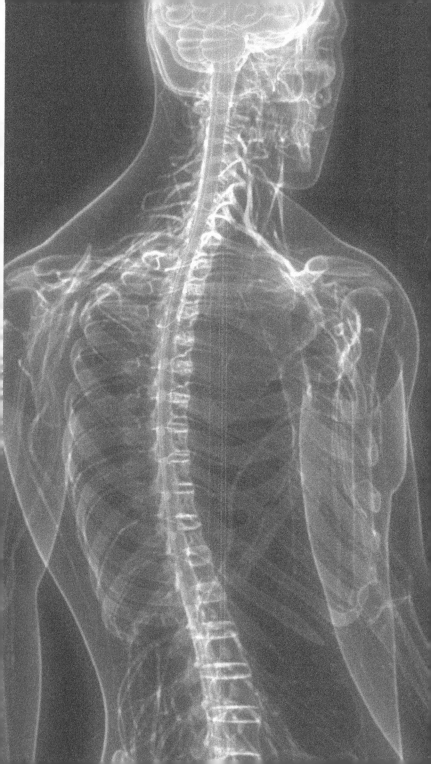

RESOURCES

Spinal Cord Injury Organizations

United Spinal Association

Dedicated to enhancing the quality of life of all people living with spinal cord injuries and disorders (SCI/D), including veterans, and providing support and information to loved ones, care providers and professionals.

(718) 803-3782
askus@unitedspinal.org

American Spinal Injury Association (ASIA)

Group of medical and other professionals engaged in treatment of spinal cord injury to promote and establish standards for health care, education, to foster research, and to facilitate communication between members.

(877) 274-2724
asia.office@asia-spinalinjury.org

Canadian American Spinal Research Organizations

Dedicated to the funding of targeted research to maximize functional recovery and cure paralysis caused by spinal cord injury. Also helps to reduce occerence spinal cord injuries through prevention and awareness programs.

(905) 508-4000
info@crso.com

Christopher & Dana Reeve Foundation

Supports research to develop effective treatments and a cure for paralysis caused by spinal cord injury. Provides a comprehensive source of information for people living with paralysis and their caregivers.

(800) 225-0292
information@christopherreeve.org

Conquer Paralysis Now

Funds scientific research, medical treatment, rehabilitation, and technological advances that lead toward a cure–whether through positive advances or failures that help guide the next effort.

(702) 463-2940
info@conquerparalysisnow.org

Craig H. Neilson Foundation

This organization is dedicated to a future where individuals with spinal cord injuries live full and productive lives as active participants in their communities.

(818) 925-1245
contact@chnfoundation.org

Hill Foundation

Offers a web resource, www.facingdisability.com, with more than 1,000 videos drawn from interviews of people with spinal cord injuries, their families, their caregivers, and experts. This is especially helpful for people who are homebound.

(312) 284-2525
info@facingdisability.com

Mike Utley Foundation

Committed to providing financial support of selected research, rehabilitation, and education programs on spinal cord injuries. It seeks financial assistance through special events, fundraising, and corporate and individual support.

(800) 294-4683

contact@mikeutley.org

Morton Cure Paralysis Fund

Dedicated to finding a cure for spinal cord injuries by raising money for spinal cord injury research. Uses a peer review process of experts to allocate funds to projects that offer the most potential for moving science forward.

(612) 904-1420
info@mcpf.org

Paralyzed Veterans of America (PVA)

Resource for veterans and for all Americans with a spinal cord injury or disease, as well as their families and the professional communities who serve them.

(800) 424-8200
info@pva.org

Spinal Cord Injury Network International

Dedicated to facilitating access to quality health care by providing information and referral services to spinal-cord-injured individuals and their families.

(800) 548-2673
spinal@sonic.net

United Spinal Association

Dedicated to enhancing the quality of life of all people living with spinal cord injuries and disorders and providing support and information to loved ones, care providers and professionals.

(718) 803-3782
askus@unitedspinal.org

Wings for Life

Provides targeted financial support, such as helping with a vehicle purchase, to enable the implementation of important research projects focusing on curing paraplegia. Also support revolutionary compensatory treatments, which promise to significantly improve the quality of life of paraplegic patients.

(310) 460-5399
office@wingsforlife.com

Model Systems Centers

From their website: The Spinal Cord Injury Model System program, sponsored by the National Institute on Disability, Independent Living, and Rehabilitation Research (NIDILRR), Office of Special Education and Rehabilitative Services, Administration for Community Living, and U.S. Department of Health and Human Services, supports innovative projects, the delivery, demonstration, and evaluation of medical, vocational, and other services to meet the needs of individuals with spinal cord injury.

Model Systems Centers across the United States work together to demonstrate improved care, maintain a national database, participate in independent and collaborative research, and provide continuing education relating to spinal cord injury. Presently, there are 14 systems and 5 follow-up centers.

Even if you went to rehab, if it wasn't sufficient and up to the standard of care, consider asking your insurance company to pay for you to go to a Model Systems Center.

Alabama
UAB Spinal Cord Injury Model System
University of Alabama at Birmingham, Birmingham, AL
(205) 934-3283

California
Southern California Spinal Cord Injury Model System
Rancho Los Amigos National Rehabilitation Center, Downey, CA
(562) 385-8111

Colorado
The Rocky Mountain Regional SCI System
Craig Hospital, Englewood, CO
(303) 789-8306

Florida
South Florida Spinal Cord Injury Model Systems
University of Miami and Jackson Memorial Hospital, Miami, FL
(305) 243-4497

Georgia
Southeastern Regional Spinal Cord Injury Model System
Shepherd Center, Atlanta, GA
(404) 352-2020

Illinois
Midwest Regional Spinal Cord Injury Care System
Shirley Ryan AbilityLab, Chicago, IL
(312) 238-2920

Massachusetts
Spaulding New England Regional Spinal Cord Injury Center
Charlestown, MA
(617) 952-6174

New Jersey
Northern New Jersey Spinal Cord Injury System
Kessler Foundation, West Orange, NJ
(973) 324-3567

New York
Mount Sinai Hospital Spinal Cord Injury Model System
Department of Rehabilitation Medicine, New York, NY
(212) 659-9369

Ohio
Northeast Ohio Regional Spinal Cord Injury System
Case Western Reserve University, Cleveland, OH
(216) 778-8781

Ohio Regional SCI Model System
Ohio State University, Wexner Medical Center, Columbus, OH
(614) 366-3877

Pennsylvania
Regional SCI Center of the Delaware Valley
Thomas Jefferson University Hospital, Philadelphia, PA
(215) 955-6579

University of Pittsburgh Model Center on Spinal Cord Injury
UMPC Rehabilitation Institute, Pittsburgh, PA
(412) 232-7949

Texas
Texas Model Spinal Cord Injury System
TIRR Memorial Hermann, Houston, TX
(713) 797-7440

Follow-Up Centers
These centers were previously funded Model Systems and
continue to collect Form II follow-up data. New participants
are not enrolled.

California
Santa Clara Valley Medical Center
San Jose, CA
(800) 352-1956

Michigan
University of Michigan
Ann Arbor, MI
(734) 763-0971

Washington
Northwest Regional Spinal Cord Injury System
University of Washington, Seattle, WA
(800) 366-5643

Accessible Gadgets and Aids

Adaptive Driving Alliance
A nationwide group of vehicle-modification dealers who provide adaptive equipment for disabled drivers and passengers.

(330) 928-7401

Amramp
A national manufacturer and supplier of wheelchair ramps and showers.

(888) 715-7598
info@amramp.com

EasyStand
This standing frame enables people with mobility-related disabilities to sit and stand. EasyStand's goal is to improve the quality of life for children and adults using wheelchairs worldwide.

(800) 343-8968

Friends of Disabled Adults and Children (FODAC)
FODAC's mission is to provide durable medical equipment (DME), such as wheelchairs and hospital beds, at little or no cost to the disabled and their families.

(770) 491-9014 or (866) 977-1204

HandiHelp.net
Website that contains simple ideas and tools that are either inexpensive to purchase or cost little to make.

handihelp@live.com

Infinitec: Infinite Potential through Technology
Infinitec provides information about assistive technology as well as training, equipment, and access to specialists and resources.

(708) 444-8460

NUPRODX INC
Shower / commode chairs and tub slider systems built for durability and portability, with a modular design that allows for adaptability to nearly any living situation, be it at home or on the road. NUPRODX is dedicated to creating innovative products to improve the lives of people who face new challenges.

(707) 934-8266
info@nuprodx.com

Paws With a Cause
Paws With a Cause enhances the independence and quality of life for people with disabilities across the national through custom-trained Assistance Dog

(616) 877-7297
paws@pawswithacause.org

University of Alabama at Birmingham Spinal Cord Injury Model System Information Network
A resource to promote knowledge in the areas of research, health, and quality of life for people with spinal cord injuries, their families, and SCI-related professionals. Includes educational materials and research. You can learn about how to participate in current trials at https://www.uab.edu/medicine/sci.

(205) 934-3283
sciweb@uab.edu

Southern California Spinal Cord Injury Model System
This system offers innovative research and education to
improve the quality of life for persons with disabilities.

(562) 385-8111
scims@ranchoresearch.org

Rocky Mountain Regional SCI System
This free-standing long-term acute care and rehabilitation
hospital provides a comprehensive system of inpatient and
outpatient medical care, rehabilitation, neurosurgical
rehabilitative care, and long-term follow up services.

Susie@craighospital.org

South Florida SCIMS
This program provides a comprehensive system of care from
the time of injury through reintegration into the community.

(305) 243-4497
efelix@miami.edu

Southeastern Regional Spinal Cord Injury Model System
A national leader in spinal cord injury care and research
under the Model Systems of Care by the U.S. Department
of Education's National Institute on Disability, Independent
Living, and Rehabilitation Research (NIDILRR).

(404) 352-2020
Edelle_Field-Fote@shepherd.org

Midwest Regional Spinal Cord Injury Care System
This leading center for innovative, integrated, interdisci-
plinary care for persons with SCI and as one of the original
five NIDILRR-designated Model System Spinal Cord Injury
Centers (in partnership with Northwestern University and

Northwestern Memorial Hospital)

(312) 238-2920
aheinemann@sralab.org

Wheelchair Distributors

21st Century Scientific, Inc.
>One of the largest wheelchair manufacturers in the world with a focus on enhancing the lifestyle of the power wheelchair user.

>(800) 448-3680

Invacare
>Groundbreaking innovations that fundamentally changed the wheelchair industry.

>(800) 333-6900

Permobil
>Leader in the complex rehabilitation power wheelchairs industry.
>(800) 736-0925

>richard.foshee@permobil.com

Pride Mobility
>A world leader in the design, development, and manufacture of mobility products–power chairs, scooters and lift chairs– for people with disabilities and mobility impairments

>(800) 522-7391
>info@pridemobility.com

Sunrise Medical
> A world leader in the development, design, manufacture, and distribution of manual wheelchairs, power wheelchairs, motorized scooters, and both standard and customized seating and positioning systems.

> (800) 333-4000
> enquiries@sunmed.co.uk

Therapeutic Activity/Adaptive Sports

Life Rolls On
> Dedicated to improving the quality of life for people living with various disabilities. Believes that adaptive surfing and skating may inspire infinite possibilities beyond any disability.

> (424) 272-1992

Move United
> Provides a list of over 40 adaptive sports, locations that offer special access, and other resources.

> (301) 217-0960
> info@moveunitedsport.org

Will2Walk Foundation
> Mission is to keep people with SCI active, fit, and independent. Aims to inspire people with SCI to achieve the highest quality of life possible.

> (480) 231-7256
> contact@will2walk

State Vocational Rehabilitation Centers

Every state has a vocational rehabilitation agency that's designed to help people with disabilities meet their employment goals. Vocational rehabilitation agencies assist individuals with disabilities to prepare for, obtain, maintain, or regain employment. The following list, from www.askearn.org/state-vocational-rehabilitation-agencies/ includes links to websites and other contact information for vocational rehabilitation (VR) agencies in the United States and its territories.

Alabama

Alabama Department of Rehabilitation Services
Phone: (334) 293-7500
Toll-Free: (800) 441-7607
Toll-Free Restrictions: AL residents
Fax: (334) 293-7383
www.rehab.alabama.gov/

Alaska

Division of Vocational Rehabilitation
Phone: (907) 465-2814
Toll-Free: (800) 478-2815
Fax: (907) 465-2856
www.labor.alaska.gov/dvr/home.htm

Arizona

Rehabilitation Services Administration
Toll-Free: (800) 563-1221
TTY: (602) 340-7771 (Maricopa County)
TTY: (855) 475-8194 (outside Maricopa County)
www.azdes.gov/rsa/

Arkansas
Rehabilitation Services Division
Phone: (501) 296-1600
Website: www.ace.arkansas.gov/arrehabservices/pages/default.aspx

Arkansas Department of Human Services
Division of Services for the Blind
Phone: (501) 682-5463
TTY: (501) 682-0093
Fax: (501) 682-0366
Wesbite: www.humanservices.arkansas.gov/dsb/pages/default.aspx

California
California Department of Rehabilitation
Phone: (916) 324-1313
TTY: (916) 558-5807
Website: www.dor.ca.gov/

Colorado
Division of Vocational Rehabilitation
Phone: (303) 866-4150,
Toll-Free: (866) 870-4595
Fax: (303) 866-4905 / (303) 866-4908
TTY: (303) 866-4150
Website: www.colorado.gov/cs/satellite/cdhs-selfsuff/
cbon/1251580884712

Connecticut
Bureau of Rehabilitation Services
Phone: (860) 424-4844
Toll-Free: (800) 537-2549
Fax: (860) 424-4850
Video Phone: (860) 920-7163
Website: www.brs.state.ct.us/

Vocational Rehabilitation Division
State Board of Education and Services for the Blind
Phone: (860) 602-4000
Toll-Free: (800) 842-4510
Fax: (860) 602-4020
TTY: (860) 602-4221
Website: www.ct.gov/besb/site/default.asp

Delaware
Division of Vocational Rehabilitation (New Castle County)
Phone: (302) 761-8275
TTY: (302) 761-8275
Website: www.dvr.delawareworks.com/

Division of Vocational Rehabilitation (Delaware)
Division for the Visually Impaired
Phone: (302) 255-9800
Fax: (302) 255-4441
Fax (eye reports only): (302) 255-9921
TTY: (302) 255-9854
Website: www.state.de.us/dhss/dvi/index.html

District of Columbia
Department on Disability Services
Phone: (202) 730-1700
Fax: (202) 730-1843
TTY: (202) 730-1516
Website: www.dds.dc.gov/

Florida
Division of Vocational Rehabilitation
Phone: (850) 245-3399
Toll-Free: (800) 451-4327
TTY: (850) 245-3399
Fax: (850) 245-3316
Website: www.rehabworks.org/

Division of Blind Services
Phone: (850) 245-0300
Toll-Free: (800) 342-1828
Fax: (850) 245-0363
Website: www.dbs.myflorida.com

Georgia
Georgia Vocational Rehabilitation Agency
Phone: (866) 489-0001
TTY: (404) 232-1998
Fax: (404) 232-1800
Website: www.gvra.georgia.gov/

Hawaii
Vocational and Rehabilitation Agency
Vocational Rehabilitation and Services for the Blind Division
Phone: (808) 586-5275
Fax: (808) 586-9755
TTY: (808) 586-5288
Website: www.hawaiivr.org/

Idaho
Division of Vocational Rehabilitation
Phone: (208) 334-3390
Website: www.vr.idaho.gov/
Vocational Rehabilitation Agency

State Commission for the Blind and Visually Impaired
Phone: (208) 334-3220
Toll-Free: (800) 542-8688
Toll-Free Restrictions: ID residents only
Fax: (208) 334-2963
Website: www.icbvi.state.id.us/

Illinois
Division of Rehabilitation Services
Toll-Free: (800) 843-6154
Toll-Free Restrictions: IL residents only
TTY: (800) 447-6404
Website: www.dhs.state.il.us/page.aspx?item=29736

Indiana
Division of Disability and Rehabilitative Services
Toll-Free: (800) 545-7763
Fax: (317) 232-1240
Website: www.in.gov/fssa/2328.htm

Iowa
Vocational Rehabilitation Services
Phone: (515) 281-4211
Fax: (515) 281-7645
TTY: (515) 281-4211
Website: www.ivrs.iowa.gov/

Vocational Rehabilitation Agency
State Department for the Blind
Phone: (515) 281-1333
Toll-Free: (800) 362-2587
Toll-Free Restrictions: IA residents only
Fax: (515) 281-1263
TTY: (515) 281-1355
Website: www.blind.iowa.gov/

Kansas
Department of Social and Rehabilitation Services
Phone: (785) 368-7471
Toll-Free: (866) 213-9079
Fax: (785) 368-7467
TTY: (785) 368-7478
Website: www.srs.ks.gov/services/Pages/Vocational.aspx

Kentucky
Kentucky Office of Vocational Rehabilitation
Phone: (502) 564-4440
Toll-Free: (800) 372-7172
Website: www.ovr.ky.gov/

Vocational and Rehabilitation Agency
State Office for the Blind
Phone: (502) 564-4754
Toll-Free: (800) 321-6668
Website: www.blind.ky.gov/

Louisiana
Rehabilitation Services State Office
Phone: (225) 219-2225
Toll-Free: (800) 737-2958
Fax: (225) 219-2942 / (225) 219-4993
Website: www.laworks.net/workforcdev/lrs/lrs_main.asp

Maine
Bureau of Rehabilitation Services
Phone: (207) 623-6799
Toll-Free: (888) 755-0023
Fax: (207) 287-5292
TTY: (888) 755-0023
Website: www.maine.gov/rehab/index.shtml

Maryland
Division of Rehabilitation Services
Phone: (410) 554-9442
Toll-Free: (888) 554-0334
Fax: (410) 554-9412
TTY: (410) 554-9411
V.P. (443) 453-5981
Website: www.dors.state.md.us/

Massachusetts
Massachusetts Rehabilitation Commission
Phone: (617) 204-3600
Toll-Free: (800) 245-6543
Fax: (617) 727-1354
TTY: (800) 245-6543
Website: www.state.ma.us/mrc/

Vocational Rehabilitation Agency
State Commission for the Blind
Phone: (617) 727-5550
Toll-Free: (800) 392-6450
Toll-Free Restrictions: MA residents only
Fax: (617) 626-7685
TTY: (800) 392-6556
Website: www.state.ma.us/mcb/

Michigan
Michigan Commission for the Blind
Phone: (517) 373-2062
Toll-Free: (800) 292-4200
Fax: (517) 335-5140
TTY: (888) 864-1212
Website: www.michigan.gov/lara/0,4601,7-154-61256_28313—,00.
html

Rehabilitation Services
Phone: (517) 373-3390
Fax: (517) 335-7277
TTY: (888) 605-6722
Website: www.michigan.gov/mdcd/0,1607,7-122-25392—,00.html

Minnesota
State Services for the Blind
Phone: (651) 642-0500
Toll-Free: (800) 652-9000
Fax: (651) 649-5927
TTY: (651) 642-0506
Website: www.mnssb.org/

Vocational Rehabilitation Services
Toll-Free: (651) 259-7114
Website: www.deed.state.mn.us/rehab/

Mississippi
Office of Vocational Rehabilitation
Toll-Free: (800) 443-1000
Website: www.mdrs.ms.gov/pages/default.aspx

Missouri
Division of Vocational Rehabilitation
Phone: (573) 751-3251
Toll-Free: (877) 222-8963
Fax: (573) 751-1441
TTY: (573) 751-0881
Website: www.dese.mo.gov/vr/

Rehabilitation Services for the Blind
Phone: (573) 751-4249
Fax: (573) 751-4984
Toll-Free: (800) 592-6004
Website: www.dss.mo.gov/fsd/rsb/index.htm

Montana
Montana Vocational Rehabilitation
Phone: (406) 444-2590
Toll-Free: (877) 296-1197
Fax: (406) 444-3632
TTY: (406) 444-2590
Website: www.dphhs.mt.gov/detd/vocrehab/

Nebraska
Nebraska Commission for the Blind and Visually Impaired
Phone: (402) 471-2891
Toll-Free: (877) 809-2419
Fax: (402) 471-3009
Website: www.ncbvi.ne.gov/

Vocational Rehabilitation
Phone: (402) 471-3644
Toll-Free: (877) 637-3422
Toll-Free Restrictions: NE residents only
Fax: (402) 471-0788
Website: www.vr.nebraska.gov/

Nevada
Rehabilitation Division (Northern Nevada)
Phone: (775) 684-4040
TTY: (775) 684-8400
Website: www.detr.state.nv.us/rehab/reh_vorh.htm

Rehabilitation Division (Southern Nevada)
Phone: (702) 486-5230
TTY: (702) 486-1018
Website: www.detr.state.nv.us/rehab/reh_vorh.htm

New Hampshire
Vocational Rehabilitation
Phone: (603) 271-3471
Toll-Free: (800) 299-1647
Fax: (603) 271-7095
Website: www.education.nh.gov/who-we-are/deputy-commissioner/bureau-of-vocational-rehabilitation

New Jersey
Commission for the Blind and the Visually Impaired
Phone: (973) 648-3333
Toll-Free: (877) 685-8878
Website: www.state.nj.us/humanservices/cbvi/home/

New Mexico
Division of Vocational Rehabilitation
Phone: (505) 954-8500 / (505) 954-8562
Toll-Free: (800) 224-7005
Website: www.dvrgetsjobs.com

New York
State Commission for the Blind and Visually Handicapped
Toll-Free: (866) 871-3000

TTY: (866) 871-6000
Website: www.ocfs.state.ny.us/main/cbvh/

Adult Career and Continuing Education Services – Vocational
Rehabilitation (ACCES-VR)
Toll-Free: (800) 222-5627
Website: www.acces.nysed.gov/vr

North Carolina

Division of Vocational and Rehabilitation Services
Toll-Free: (800) 689-9090
Fax: (919) 733-7968
TTY: 919-855-3579
VP: (919) 324-1500
Website: www.dvr.dhhs.state.nc.us/

North Dakota

Division of Vocational Rehabilitation
Phone: (701) 328-8950
Toll-Free: (800) 755-2745
Fax: (701) 328-8969
Website: www.nd.gov/dhs/dvr/index.html

Ohio

Bureau of Vocational Rehabilitation
Phone: (614) 438-1200
Website: www.ood.ohio.gov/

Oklahoma

Oklahoma Department of Rehabilitation Services
Phone: (405) 951-3400
Toll-Free: (800) 845-8476
TTY: (405) 951-3400 / (800) 845-8476
Website: www.okrehab.org/

Oregon
Office of Vocational Rehabilitation Services
Phone: (503) 945-5880
Toll-Free: (877) 277-0513
Fax: (503) 947-5010
Website: www.oregon.gov/dhs/vr/

Pennsylvania
Office of Vocational Rehabilitation
Phone: (717) 787-5244
Toll-Free: (800) 442-6351
TTY: (717) 787-4885 / (866) 830-7327
Website: www.dli.pa.gov/individuals/disability-services/ovr/
pages/ovr-office-directory.aspx

Blindness and Visual Services
Phone: (717) 787-6176
Toll-Free: (800) 622-2842
TTY: (717) 787-4885
TTY (2): (866) 830-7327
Website: www.dli.pa.gov/individuals/disability-services/bbvs/
pages/default.aspx

Rhode Island
Vocational and Rehabilitation Agency
Phone: (401) 421-7005
TTY: (401) 421-7016
Website: www.ors.state.ri.us

South Carolina
South Carolina Vocational Rehabilitation Department
Phone: (803) 896-6500 (Columbia area)
Toll-Free: (800) 832-7526
TTY: (803) 896-6553
Website: www.scvrd.net/

South Dakota
Division of Rehabilitation Services
Phone: (605) 773-3195
Fax: (605) 773-5483
Website: www.dhs.sd.gov/drs/

Tennessee
Vocational Rehabilitation Services
Phone: (615) 313-4891
Fax: (615) 741-6508
TTY: (615) 313-5695 / (800) 270-1349
Website: www.tn.gov/humanservices/ds/vocational-rehabilitation.html

Texas
Department of Assistive and Rehabilitative Services
Toll-Free: (800) 628-5115
TTY: (866) 581-9328
Website: www.dars.state.tx.us/

Utah
Utah State Office of Rehabilitation
Phone: (801) 538-7530
Toll-Free: (800) 473-7530
Fax: (801) 538-7522
TTY: (801) 538-7530
Website: www.usor.utah.gov/

Vermont
Vocational Rehabilitation
Phone: (802) 241-1455
Toll-Free: (866) 879-6757
TTY: (802) 241-1455
Website: www.vocrehab.vermont.gov/

Virginia
Department of Rehabilitation Services
Phone: (804) 662-7000
Toll-Free: (800) 552-5019
Fax: (804) 662-9532
TTY: (800) 464-9950
Website: www.vadrs.org/

Washington
Division of Vocational Rehabilitation
Phone: (360) 725-3636
Toll-Free: (800) 637-5627
Fax: (360) 438-8007
TTY: (800) 637-5627 / (360) 725-3636
Website: www.dshs.wa.gov/dvr/

Department of Services for the Blind (DSB)
Phone: (800) 552-7103
Website: www.dsb.wa.gov/

West Virginia
Division of Rehabilitation Services
Phone: (304) 356-2060
Toll-Free: (800) 642-8207
Website: www.wvdrs.org/

Wisconsin
Division of Vocational Rehabilitation
Phone: (608) 261-0050
Toll-Free: (800) 442-3477
Fax: (608) 266-1133
TTY: (888) 877-5939
Website: www.dwd.wisconsin.gov/dvr

Wyoming
Division of Vocational Rehabilitation
Phone: (307) 777-8650
Fax: (307) 777-5857
Website: www.wyomingworkforce.org/pages/default.aspx

U.S. Territories

American Samoa
Division of Vocational Rehabilitation
Phone: (684) 699-1371 / (684) 699-4234
Website: www.americansamoa.gov/index.php/2012-04-25-19-44-32/2012-04-28-01-30-33/offices/2012-04-30-18-53-34

Commonwealth of the Northern Mariana Islands
CNMI Office of Vocational Rehabilitation
Phone: (670) 322-6537
Fax: (670) 322-6536
TTY: (670) 322-6449
Website: www.ovrgov.net

Guam
Division of Vocational Rehabilitation
Phone: (671) 642-0022
Website: www.dol.guam.gov/index.php?option=com_
content&view=article&id=115:department-of-integrated-
services-for-individuals-with-disabilities&catid=82:
division-of-vocational-rehabilitation&Itemid=182

Puerto Rico
Vocational Rehabilitation Administration
Phone: (787) 729-0160
Fax: (787) 728-8070
TTY: (787) 268-3735
Website: www.gobierno.pr/gprportal/inicio

U.S. Virgin Islands
Division of Disabilities and Rehabilitation Services
Phone: (340) 774-0930 ext. 4190
Fax: (340) 774-7773
TTY: (340) 776-2043
Website: www.dhs.gov.vi/disabilities/index.html

Acknowledgments

This book is a labor of love for other people with spinal cord injury. Without the experiences and support from my SCI peers, this book would not exist. I hope this book helps you avoid the mistakes I made and find resources to live your best life.

Writing a book is harder and more rewarding than I could have ever imagined. None of this would have been possible without my friend Martha. Thank you for standing by me in good times and bad. You are an angel.

There are so many people to thank. First, thank you to my family for their love and support. You understand it all. I love you very much!

Jennifer and everyone at Bright Communications, your kindness, generosity, and assistance made this book possible. Thank you for the encouragement.

My mentors Dr. Bob Collins; Dr. Bruce Dobkin; John Mazziotta, MD, PhD; and the UCLA Family that has given me support throughout most of my spinal cord injury, you kept me Pushing Forward. Thank you for the never-ending encouragement.

Brooke, Paul, and Gary, the best friends in the world, are always there for me when things get tough. Thanks for holding me up.

The world is a better place thanks to people who want to develop and lead others. What makes it even better are people who share the gift of their time to mentor future leaders. Thank you to Draion Burch, who strives to grow and help others grow.

I want to thank *everyone* who said anything positive to me or taught me something. MMA21 I heard it all and it meant something.

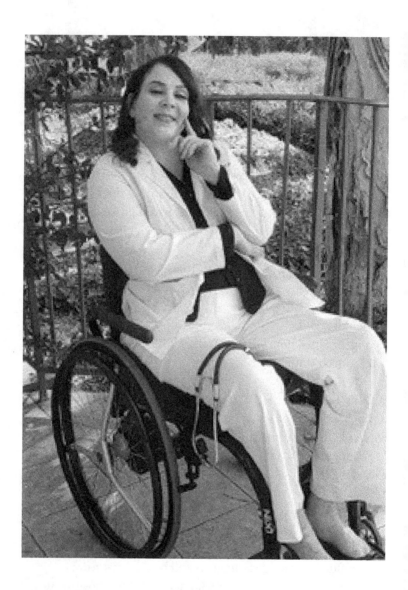

About the Author

Susan Douglas, MD, JD, knows persistence and perseverance. Dr. Douglas was 21 when her car skidded off the road. In less than a year, she returned to Georgetown University Medical School a paraplegic, where she was a trailblazer. In 1996, she began practicing academic neurology medicine at UCLA, combining lab research, clinical medicine, and teaching. Changes in healthcare and insight from her own experiences motivated her move toward public policy and the law. She received her law degree at Westhaven University in Cypress, California, in 2008.

Dr. Douglas fights barriers wherever she finds them. Her struggle with provisions such as the Medicare Homebound Rule, Community First Choice, and other regulations that essentially block access to independence all drive her passion to change healthcare policy. She strives to be an effective advocate, thought leader, coalition builder, and solution driver, for public and private entities that are affected by healthcare-policy.

She focuses on reducing disparities, ending discrimination, promoting equality of opportunity, and employment for under-represented groups and civil human rights. Dr. Douglas believes that everyone shares essentially the same daily struggles, victories, and defeats, regardless of occupation or social status.

"We all benefit when these struggles and outcomes are acknowledged and validated. We are all one people in the same boat, fighting the same fight," she says.

Currently, Dr. Douglas is an adjunct assistant professor of neurology at UCLA Department of Neurology.

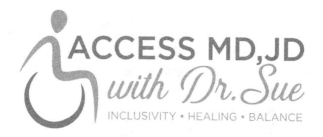

ACCESS MD,JD
with Dr. Sue
INCLUSIVITY • HEALING • BALANCE

After 35 years of living with and treating spinal cord injury, I am moving on to help people adapt to the experience of spinal cord injury. I've created Access MD, JD to help new spinal cord injured and their families navigate the confusing, corporate health care terrain. No one ever thinks a tragedy like a spinal cord injury will happen to them. You're in shock, and you don't know what to do. The purpose of Access MD, JD is to help you make decisions during this tragic time by sharing my experiences and what I wish I would have known to help make your experience easier and to help you continue to live your best life.

Through Access MD, JD, I offer my consulting services, including help with grief, mindset, family dynamics, medical decision making, financial and legal advice, support services, and home modification suggestions. I'm available for individual consulting, small groups, and workshop and conference speaking engagements.

For more information, contact info@DrSueMDJD.com.

CPSIA information can be obtained
at www.ICGtesting.com
Printed in the USA
LVHW050546260621
691140LV00012B/1836